CONVERSATIONS
with a PRINCE

CONVERSATIONS
with a PRINCE

A YEAR OF RIDING
AT EAST HILL FARM

HELEN HUSHER

THE LYONS PRESS
Guilford, Connecticut
An imprint of The Globe Pequot Press
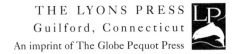

To buy books in quantity for corporate use
or incentives, call **(800) 962–0973, ext. 4551,**
or e-mail **premiums@GlobePequot.com.**

The Lyons Press is an imprint of The Globe Pequot Press

10 9 8 7 6 5 4 3 2 1

Printed in the United States of America

Designed by Lisa Reneson

ISBN 1-59228-693-3

Library of Congress Cataloging-in-Publication data is available on file.

TO CAROLINE

good with horses

acknowledgments

Special thanks go out to my teacher, Kathie Moulton, and to Jeanette Hogan, Ruth Hogan-Poulsen, Gina Dimick, Con Hogan, Bill Moulton, and all the students and barn staff at East Hill Farm. Without them, not a word of this book would have been possible. These fine people let me hang around, eavesdrop, and ask questions so long as I also did some stalls and helped with the noon watering.

For his support, affection, and ongoing belief that the book would please a general, nonhorsey audience, much love and much owed to my partner, Vince Sondej.

To my foster parents, Alice and Tony Pickman, a bottomless love for giving me not just a home but my beloved and exasperating horse, and for acting as if that was no big deal. It was.

For unexpected validation, thanks to my agent, Christina Ward, who took up riding after reading this manuscript and can now gossip with me about Puck and Rainbow. For background material, thanks to all the brave and tolerant animals who do not appear in these pages but who have enriched my life and explained the rules—Quinque, New Era, Juanita, Rose, and Tina, to say nothing of the only gelding I ever really loved, the consistent and indomitable Luke.

And finally, thanks to all the usual suspects—my teachers Alex Gold and Celia Millward, and my friend Alfred Perry who said to me, almost in passing, that it would please him if someday I might write a book. "About what?" I asked. "It doesn't matter," he replied. "Just write one. I'd like that."

CONVERSATIONS
with a PRINCE

ONE

EVER SINCE MY EARLY TEENS, MY OFF-THE-RACK ANXIETY dream has always been that I have left my horse standing forgotten in the cross ties. While not a felony, this is definitely a crime, and when I mentioned this to Kathie she responded with a little laugh, maybe because she recognized the dream or maybe because other people's worries often seem faintly ridiculous. "If you left Prince in the cross ties," she said, "I think somebody would notice and put him up for you."

Kathie Moulton is a co-owner and teacher at East Hill Farm, a thirty-horse boarding and lesson barn set into the shoulder of a ridge in Plainfield, Vermont. Despite the name, the farm actually faces west, and if you stand at the main entrance to the barn you can see the ragged blue profile of the Worcester Range of the Green Mountains—Burnt Mountain, White Rock Mountain, Hunger Mountain. These plain, honest names seem part of the reality that no one at East Hill has the leisure to admire this view, what with all the work that must be done. For long stretches of the day, East Hill is a moving scrum of working students, regular students, staff, owners, boarders, 4-Hers, adult amateur riders, disabled riders, parents, siblings, spouses, and hangers-on; stalls are being cleaned and horses are being turned out, brought in, groomed, and spoken to; the indoor arena is full of movement, and the chalkboard near the doorway is covered with scribbled instructions about feeding, vets, and cell phones; the aisles are festooned with animals, wheelbarrows, grooming kits, horse rugs, tack, and radios. The horses who are not being worked press their long noses against the bars of their box stalls, sniff, and keep detailed minutes of the proceedings. Kathie's quite right—if I really did drive off and leave Prince standing in the cross ties, he wouldn't be allowed to stay there for long. Someone would move him just to get him out of the way.

But there is a tidal quality to the activity in a horse barn, which means there are also times at East Hill when the place is utterly still except for the sigh of horses, the rustle of bedding, and the occasional bang of a bored inhabitant kicking the wall. The effect is a little eerie: It is as if the entire cast has been vaporized by space rays or sent en masse on some urgent errand in a neighboring state. Even the bony tortoiseshell barn cat, who spends his waking hours supervising from the hayloft, is mysteriously missing; a different cat, plumper and less managerial, sleeps in a tight spiral on the heater in the tack room, and the entire barn lapses into a ghostly and peaceful deadness. You can browse in silence, visiting with each animal, and stand in the doorway and look at the mountains. The aisle is swept and some of the horses are snoozing, their noses on their folded forelegs and their leaflike ears at half-mast. The depth of this silence, and the fact that the animals all know how to make use of it, tells me that East Hill is a well-run place.

It was on one of these quiet days in midwinter that I was sent to get Prince out of the paddock for my lesson. East Hill Farm, as an institution, believes firmly in regular turnout—it keeps horses socialized and calm—and this means that the animals are often inconveniently spaced and slightly grubby. I wasn't wearing my glasses, but I'd been told Prince was the one wearing a green rug and that he was a buckskin, and even in a blurry world this should have been plenty of identification. As I crunched through the snow toward the gate, though, all I could see were two leggy balls of mud, one large and one small, who hung together like a pair of adolescents sneaking cigarettes at the far end of the fence line. The larger ball looked at me, snorted a little, and told the smaller ball a disrespectful joke, and then they both turned to see what I would do. The two of them looked like the aftermath of the worst kind of fraternity gathering—the smaller ball didn't really even have a rug on anymore, since it had slipped across his back and down, and it dragged on the ground like a mammoth bib. The larger one was mostly just caked, but he'd done a good job of it, and there seemed to be a blob of topsoil drying in a knob on the top of his head. They both looked dissolute and dirty and vaguely delinquent. I hoped, fervently, that the larger horse was Prince, mostly because there was something about the level of alert scrutiny coming off the smaller horse that told me he probably had a pony temperament. Ponies are fine for small people who don't mind jokes being made at their expense, but I'm big and sometimes take things personally. The larger horse looked far more normal; he'd managed to remain properly dressed and had a generically pretty outline. Chipping off the mud to find the hair color underneath, I discovered that Prince was of course the little one. The larger horse noted my disappointment and stuck up for his friend by inserting himself between us.

Prince, I learned in time, had a powerful gift for dishevelment. He was—is—a plain, common little creature with a blocky head, a flat top line, and a tendency toward discombobulation, so my first encounter with him was not just a fluke of the dismal Vermont winter. But grooming a really dirty horse has its satisfactions, and grooming a light-colored horse in this condition is on a par with peeling wallpaper that really wants to come off the wall. You get filthy but things happen fast—a curry loosens everything up, and a dandy brush, which looks like a long-bristled scrubbing brush, scratches through the crust to find the shape of the animal underneath. But the real joy of grooming well lies in the details—the insides of the hind legs, the improbably large but tender acreage of the underbelly, the base of the ears, the face, the chin, and the interesting and often very grubby six square inches at the back of the fetlock joint, just above the heels. These secondary and intimate destinations have always attracted me—they are complicated and not always visited often enough—and there are days when I go overboard and find myself carefully washing and drying each hard, heavy foot and dreamily inspecting the triangular, rubbery organ that protrudes from the sole, a strange evolutionary design solution that is called—clumsily—a frog.

One of the sayings in the horse world is that a clean horse is a happy horse, but in my experience this is not really true. Horses like dirt, and go to considerable trouble to burrow around in as much of it as they can find. But what horses do like is to be *tended*, and I think this is what the old saw points to: Being touched and noticed and having their parts inspected and admired puts them in a good mood. Some horses will tell you they don't like it by twitching and rolling their eyes and making objections, but this is usually because they don't like being worked, and horses tend to be groomed right before they are ridden. This contaminates what ought to be a pleasant interaction for everybody.

Prince initially approached being groomed with a generic tolerance, maintaining an amenable silence on the general topics of having his feet picked out and the curry applied. He also refrained from making any of the usual faces, but, apart from a bit of wrigglyness, his policy on being groomed was that it was a thing that was done *to* him; he didn't need to participate. He seemed to ignore me and looked out the barn door at nothing in particular. His barn manners were good, and this is not a common thing in a lesson horse, a creature ridden often and hard by a lot of different people who all make mistakes, some of them painful, and many of them hard to anticipate. His goodness impressed me, but I failed to make much of an impression in return.

What got Prince's attention was my love of detailing. As I brushed out his thick toothbrush of a mane, carefully separating out the scurf and resolving the tangles, he turned and looked at me cautiously, pleased but uncertain—because his mane is dense and formidable, it's possible this didn't happen all that often. When I also lingered over his thick, oily tail, he shifted his haunches and swung his head several times so he could see me clearly. By the time I was ready to approach his ears and face with a soft brush and a cloth, he was following my movements with accumulating interest, as if I might be mildly but pleasantly deranged.

Grooming a horse's face is intimate; it involves acceptance and trust in a human caress. Eyes are delicate, so there is always a strong impulse to protect them by putting them up out of reach, and the lips and ears can be pinched and injured with amazing ease. Because of this, face grooming must proceed as if there is all the time in the world, which there almost never is—lessons must begin on time and schedules honored—but you can't let even a corner of that hurried reality intrude. Prince, after a few preliminary protective measures, suddenly proved more than ready for a long dalliance while I brushed and wiped and used my fingertips to tease the dried dribble from the corners of his eyes. Sighing happily, he deposited his chin on my shoulder and thudded his lips together; when I began the careful work around his ears, he tipped his ugly head toward me and momentarily buried his face in the front of my jacket. By the time I began on his chin and throatlatch, he was helping me in every way he could think of, tipping and lifting so I could work on the deep groove between his lower jaws that led to the wrinkly knob of his chin, and when I wiped the crud out of his nose he smacked his lips and showed me his oblong tongue.

I had come back to horses after seven years away—I'd off-loaded my last one during a divorce and, because that experience was painful, hadn't seriously touched one since. In the time that had flickered by, I'd been busy with an interesting job, a new partner, and writing a couple of books. I told myself—often, and with stoicism—that once I had gone beyond fifty there was really no call for me to be putting myself at risk by hanging around large, powerful creatures who were not always predictable. What's more, I told myself—often—I really wasn't in the market for anything that was likely to drain away my small supply of money.

But during one sunny, crinkly autumn, I had ridden out over several days with my foster sister and niece along the seashore in southern Massachusetts, and even though I had made this same ride a dozen times before on previous visits, this one seemed different. I had been acquired as a young teenager by a large and very talkative family, and usually these long hacks on borrowed horses tended to be social engagements: We would get up on a trail along the shoulder of a hill, enjoy the long views across Vineyard Sound, and gossip. This time around, we talked about our parents, who were getting old, and what to worry about, and whether there was anything that ought to be done, and we talked about my sister's new house in Rhode Island and her neighbors and her job; we talked about my plans to move from one town in central Vermont to another, and about whether I wanted to get a dog. Dogs, we decided, could be a real pain; cats were easier, but cats were never particularly glad to see you. "I miss Tilly and Lucius," Caroline said, rather suddenly. "I think I'd rather have Tilly and Lucius back than all the dogs in the world." Tilly and Lucius were a pair of horses she'd had in England, where she lived for more than a decade, and there was something in the way she said this that was hot and sharp and instantly painful. It made me think that the good-enough life, the life I'd chosen, was looking a little empty.

I was primed to think this because, a few weeks before, I'd dragged my partner, Vince, to a nearby horse show. We'd ridden there on his motorcycle—a near-vintage, rumbling machine that I had come to view with considerable joy. It not only made a nice sound—a rich, happy, mechanical purring—but also woke up the senses. On a motorcycle, the things in the world around you seem abnormally real: When you enter the shade, not only does the temperature drop and make bumps on your skin, but you can feel the thick forest pumping out new air with a settled, treelike efficiency. You can smell water before you see it—a bluish, metallic flavor on the back of the tongue—and the brisk rows of corn by the road seem militant and sexual, ready for war. One day, riding down a road in Marshfield, I smelled pancakes. There were no pancakes anywhere to be seen, but the odor was unmistakable—there is some crop or weed or roadside flora that, at least briefly, imitates breakfast. I loved riding on the back of the bike, and secretly yearned to ride in front, but the mechanics of shifting the thing looked pretty formidable.

The horse show was, mostly, a mere destination; when there's a motorcycle in the family, you feel a need to invent places to go on it. But I also really wanted to go. As we approached the grounds, I felt the familiar tension, the rising sensation in my stomach, that meant I was going to see attractive horses do difficult things under stressful conditions. Even if I am not riding, I still have receptors for the high, electric hum of competition, with its buzzing mix of fear, hope, and validation. Prizes would be awarded, and these prizes meant something; before the end of the long day, someone would be happy and someone else would be in secret tears. Horse shows have this emotional density, and after I quit competing I actually looked into whether I could apprentice to be a horse-show judge, just so that I could keep going on the weekends. I learned that my temperament wasn't right for it—I didn't want to be responsible for hurt feelings—but I did, for a while, do fairly regular stints as an assistant to the judge, gatekeeper, and ribbon-runner, serving as one of the endless volunteers needed to make a large, complicated event run smoothly. I would get a sunburn and return home covered with fine dust, my head full of movies of horses coming endlessly down a line of fences, their tails curved away from their firm fannies, their toes tapping the wood rails with a delicate sound that I found familiar, emotionally correct, and soothing.

This particular show was A-rated, which meant that the horses were of good quality and the competition pretty stiff, but it still had all the elements that can be found in any local backyard event—the milling around, the elegant and slightly snobby riding clothes, the quacks from the loudspeaker, the whinnies of separated friends. This sameness is unshakable: Even at top shows, there are unraveling braids and crabby mothers and droopy lawn chairs set up next to coolers in the scanty shade. People at horse shows often look a little below par from getting up so early and having so much to do, but the horses themselves gleam with potential—they assume a certain horse-show aura that can best be summed up by a judge I had once assisted. Each time a horse entered the ring to jump, she said, quietly but still out loud, "This one's the one. This one will be the winner." Until the horse made the first mistake, she believed with all her heart that this was so. I liked this; it captured the essence of competition. Even standing around the gate doing nothing in particular, just waiting their turn in the ring, the animals seem almost transcendent. Anything can happen. The schooling problems and disobediences from home may have somehow vanished in the trailer, and a perfect trip over eight fences suddenly seems possible, fraught with hope and meaning. I liked working for this judge. Not only was she a good judge—she must have been, since the results from her scorecards sometimes surprised me—but she gave her work a level of attention that was nearly religious.

Vince tolerated our day at the horse show pretty well, which made me grateful. I've discovered that most people are deeply and thoroughly bored by these gatherings—to them, it's perfectly obvious that the same thing is happening over and over and over again. And in a way they are right. If you don't know where to point your attention, it really looks like the same brown horse is jumping the same obstacles in the same order for hours on end in a relentless purgatory of nothingness and dust. I understand this boredom, since I suffer from it during car chases at the movies. I can't tell these chases apart, and I don't want to, and I do not care about the outcomes, only that the outcomes arrive swiftly so the movie can resume. But car chases just keep on happening, all the time, and without my permission. The rapt attention of the people around me only reinforces my impatience and heightens my sense of my own abnormality.

But Vince was almost interested—almost. Or at least he was interested in finding out why it interested me, which is not quite the same thing, but it was more than enough to carry us through one horse show, so I explained to him the difference between an equitation class, where the rider was being judged, and a performance class, where the horse was. But I also tried to articulate that it was the horse-and-rider combination that really mattered, and that the nicest horse on the grounds could not win a performance class without a skilled rider, and the best rider could not get far in equitation without at least an adequate horse. It was one of those blurry things that just happened to be true. "So," he asked with an air of genuine inquiry, "the performance and the equitation—is it a distinction without a difference?"

"It may be," I said, surprised by his willingness to take the horse show seriously.

Riding home on the back of the motorcycle, it seemed to me again that the world was busy being beautiful. The long days of summer bring slanting sunshine at the end, and there were bars of light across the road that flickered as we broke through them; the Mad River, running alongside us for a while, had a stately, painted quality like something from the Hudson River School. Even the main street of Waterbury seemed excessively dramatic, dressed up with boxes of blue shadow and stars of sunlight bouncing off the windows. I watched our reflection in the storefronts and thought, not for the first time, that we made a nice-looking couple, casual together but confident, both large people with long, expressive arms. There was also something about our storefront reflection that made me revisit being in my early fifties, which at that moment seemed no longer past it but somehow firmly in the middle. It occurred to me that I could still have new things—a new partner, new sensations, new adventures. I had a lot to be pleased about but that night, climbing into bed, I suddenly found myself yearning for an old thing—specifically another show, with its cadence and its repetition. As I thanked Vince again for coming with me, I felt momentarily desolated, homesick for a world in which horses are groomed, braided, bandaged, and led up ramps into six-stall vans, vans with full hay nets in each narrow stall, hanging with an innocence that would be gone by the end of the day. "Why are you crying?" Vince asked.

"I want it back," I said, not really even knowing what I meant.

TWO

M Y LESSON BEGAN AND PRINCE WAS EVERYTHING I HAD imagined—choppy, spry, and eager to pursue an opportunistic pony agenda. He trotted around merrily, his short neck set against me and his midsection bulging wildly in all directions; I discovered quickly that it was nothing for him to point himself in one direction while proceeding speedily in another. The effect was entertaining, but curiously mechanical: He reminded me of a bumper car, with its yawing, mushy, and approximate steering, but his tiny strides also felt dry and strangely inanimate, as if I were mounted on a manic and perhaps defective sewing machine.

Yet Kathie insisted that Prince could, with the right rider, really do things—come into the bridle, straighten, and listen carefully, assuming I had something coherent and interesting to say. While she explained this, we skittered and sifted around together and Prince offered up a wayward gleefulness that genuinely impressed me. He had half a dozen ways of saying *no*, all of them honed to perfection but, amazingly, none of them seeming resentful or dangerous. This was Prince's comic routine, his schtick, and his basic cheerfulness about everything meant that I believed

Kathie: Prince clearly knew exactly what he was doing, and his composure and lack of malice were weirdly reassuring.

Riding lessons sound very strange, like a rap song from a planet of confirmed lunatics: "Say no to that outside shoulder," said Kathie, "and don't allow him to escape like that. No. No. No. That's it. There. No. No. No. Use that outside rein and half-halt, make it clear, now wait for his answer. No. That's too much correction. More go, he's not coming off your inside leg. That's better. Ahh—but see there you dropped him again and he popped to the outside and then you had to do two or three big things to get him back. What we want is to get rid of the big things and have little things all the time. Now don't accept that from him. Hah! Good. Better. But you still had to do too much, you still had to get in there with the big fix. No. No. No. Yes! Now there you had him, and that's what you have to sustain, but you can't be lazy and quit riding and think everything's fine. No. No. No. Look, if you need to spank him, spank him, but he can't feel you asking him and not do *something*, he has to do something, he's not allowed to tune you out. No. No. Yes. Now there's a nice answer, can you feel that? Can you? Now you're giving too much again. No. No. No. Better there, but that time it wasn't enough. Too much, then not enough. You're not making it possible for him to understand you, and you think you're being polite but he doesn't think so. That's better. No. No. No. Now here he's getting crooked because you gave away that outside hand again, because you want to be nice and this way he can avoid you, but you have to get in there and really fix it. So left flexion now. Flex left. Really flex. Pull on the left rein. Pull, and get it over with. Left. Left. Good. He's done fighting you, so now release. Always the correction, then the release. Keep up your end of things. No. No. You just abandoned him. No. No. No."

We pay money for this.

The problem was that I had no clear idea what Kathie was really talking about, since I had no picture in my mind of the result I was aiming for. This was entirely my own fault, since I'd spent most of my riding life cantering around in big fields and jumping whatever I found there—hay bales, poles held up by kitchen chairs, sawhorses, barrels, and, as I got better at it, gates, oxers, ditches, banks, and obstacles made from artfully arranged telephone poles. I had alternated this with just enough simple schooling on the flat so that my horse could lengthen and shorten stride, change a lead, turn in the air over a fence, and get presentable transitions—all necessary skills for any horse who is ever going to amount to anything. Before passing a licensing exam to be a riding teacher, I did learn a little more about riding that was not jumping, mostly because I had to be able to execute some very simple sideways movements for the riding part of the test, but once I passed my exam I went back to cantering around in the field. This kind of riding looks hard—you go fast, and there can be a lot of drama if things go wrong—but there's actually a fairly simple intellectual rhythm to it. The horse has to agree with you that it's fun, and both of you need a certain amount of courage, and the tempo of the whole enterprise has to be perfectly balanced between too much danger and too much safety.

But I was not going to be allowed to indulge in any of these monkeyshines on Prince. This was, to a large degree, Ruth's fault. Ruth—Ruth Hogan-Poulsen—is the daughter of East Hill's other co-owners, Con and Jeanette Hogan, and Ruth's success as an event rider, an equitation champion, and finally a national dressage figure seems to color the air that hangs over East Hill. Each spring, after a season in a warmer climate, Ruth pulls into the driveway with a huge horse van and discharges her students, her dogs, and her spectacular, big-fronted horses. Everything about these horses is a rebuke to my history of happy galloping. They carry themselves with power and care, as if they know that they are something to contend with; even the younger, less developed horses have an air of studiousness, perhaps because they will soon be cramming for the tests at the Intermediaire and Prix St. Georges.

This foreign-sounding terminology will not mean much to a lot of people—dressage is often spoken with a funny accent. What these words mostly convey is that these creatures, in cahoots with Ruth, are aspiring to do dressage about as well as it can be done. This is saying something, because dressage is so hard that there are times when you wonder if it's actually worth doing, even though it is. Watching a horse do dressage, especially at the higher levels, is a little bit like watching a gymnast working on the uneven bars. It's controlled, and you can tell that the gymnast has practiced like the dickens to get to this point, but to the spectator it looks both wild and curiously easy. The more skilled the gymnast, the easier it looks—it has the miraculous remembered fluidity of childhood, a time when all daring and demented things were possible and you could go down whole flights of steep stairs without actually touching them and fling yourself without injury off the high, pumping arc of the swings. This is why, when the gymnast offers that magical pause, when she does that handstand—an amazing display of strength and balance and concentration and artistry, her feet pointed at the high, lit ceiling—it is simply impossible to take your eyes away. You have to see what happens next, which way she falls, how she folds, whether she swings again or lifts her tapered legs in that impossible V and clears the lower bar. Dressage done well is exactly like this—improbable and riveting—and dressage done well also looks amazingly easy. Except it isn't. Dressage is hard.

East Hill is infused with a deeply felt commitment to this kind of riding, to the point where it has percolated down even unto the ugliest school pony. Prince obviously knew a lot more about all this stuff than I did, and his policy was that no round, engaged, or athletic movements would be forthcoming until I had earned them. In the meantime, he had a wide repertoire of other things that I could react to, most of them slovenly and uncomfortable. The fact that I could have made him go fast and jump things if I wanted to did not count for much that day, mostly because these were not things we were doing or were likely to do anytime soon. I was going to have to put Prince in the bridle, and that was that.

There is a strange, beautiful grammar to a riding lesson, and this is true even when not much gets accomplished. The cascade of words tumbling from the instructor is a nutrient medium, like that orange stuff in the bottom of a petri dish, and one of the duties of a riding teacher is to say the same things again and again, always a little differently, always rephrased and re-metaphored, so that many versions of the same idea swim in the rider's brain. On the other side of the equation is the rider, who tries out different parts of these phrases to see what might happen—a tentative and approximate process—and, if something good comes of the effort, and the phrase is heard often enough, then the teacher's metaphors slowly lose their linguistic shape and become tiny muscle memories that do not need to be talked about anymore. Yet the most interesting element in the transaction is that there is a critical third party who can only be consulted obliquely, and only after the cascade of language has been funneled into the rider and the words taken out. This third party, the horse, only knows that sometimes the rider is doing things a little differently, or is doing the same things more insistently, or is perhaps overwhelmed and doing nothing much at all. Whatever the status of all that, and whatever its various permutations, it is a transaction that requires that two participants out of three must be utterly silent.

This silence can be a little pathological—I, for one, cannot talk at all when I'm trying to ride seriously; there is something about the syncopation of the horse that makes me linguistically numb, as if I have tossed back a beakerful of novocaine. It really is a dentist-office sensation—a throbbing, drooling muteness—and I once had a teacher who was quite sure I was an idiot, since I couldn't answer his questions or even explain why I couldn't answer them. Before my first lesson began, I tried to warn Kathie about this, but I was already mounted and naturally put it badly.

"I don't talk on the horse," I said. "It's hard. I can't say things."

Kathie looked pleased. "Good," she said. "I guess that means you won't argue with me."

"I won't anything. Something is broken about talking."

"Suits me fine," she said. "Too many people do far too much talking around here anyway."

Kathie is a short woman with considerable presence, blessed with the necessary brisk authority that makes it possible to teach people and horses to behave themselves. She has a certain Mighty Mouse quality—small, fierce, and morally upright—and the good riding teacher's brisk, flexible, and reiterative command of language. Right from the first lesson, I was genuinely surprised by the density of information pouring from her, her ability to make short, detailed observations, her insistence I ride every step—early lessons generally tend to be looser, less demanding, and more evaluative, a feeling-out process. There was, of course, the Prince factor—his commitment to crookedness kept us all pretty busy—but I got the distinct and correct impression that this cascade of talkiness was Kathie's natural mode. It isn't really bossiness, although it sometimes feels bossy; it's more like a firm and palpable intensity that adds weight to the proceedings. I frankly can't imagine Kathie ever doing what I did when I was teaching, which was to disguise drills as games and corrections as mere suggestions. ("When she does that, try sending her on. If she's busy going forward, it's likely she won't have time to buck.") Would Kathie endorse my past use of an egg and spoon as a way of encouraging steadiness? If so, would she lower the stakes and hard-boil the eggs first? I doubted it.

As I got off and ran my stirrups up, I looked at Prince. He was once again in a generic, neutral mode, but there was also something vaguely self-regarding about the set of his ears, as if he'd successfully stolen a cookie. I hadn't found the lesson particularly demoralizing or unpleasant, but it was clear he had enjoyed himself more than I had; I was damp and tired while he was fresh, dry, and complacent. As I stripped him, brushed him, and reapplied his grimy rug, I found myself admiring his combination of self-assurance and intractability. I liked him, and before I left the barn I specifically asked to ride Prince again.

THREE

T HE IDEA THAT RIDING IS FOR RICH FOLKS IS BOTH TRUE AND untrue, and this is one of the things I like about the sport. Statistics compiled by the American Horse Council indicate that horses actually move more money around in the economy than the motion-picture industry, furniture and fixtures, and the U.S. rail system. The overall economic impact pegs in at $122 billion, finishing just behind textiles, clothing, and tobacco. But it's a weird sort of economy: A lot of money changes hands, but for the most part no money is actually *made*; buying a horse is not an investment so much as it is a down payment, with more bills for hay, grain, shoes, vet care, equipment, and entry fees to quickly follow. Untold thousands of dollars can be spent chasing after a piece of ribbon with a street value of perhaps twenty cents. Rodeo riders are a little farther up the wage scale with their championship saddles and belt buckles, but even at Pimlico or Churchill Downs money is being squandered at a pace that far outstrips the value of the winning purses. So in that sense, riding really is for people who can afford it. When Lewis Lapham sneers in *Harper's* about the "equestrian class," it's fun to sneer right along with him. I know what he means by this phrase, and the meaning is narrow: The equestrian class—an old Roman term for the mounted nobility—does not muck stalls, stack hay, or haul water. They hire people to do those things, often people like me, and representatives of the clan can sometimes be seen standing by the mounting block, tapping a crop against an elegant boot, waiting for a groomed animal to magically appear. But these boot-tappers are actually rare, and in my experience they are delicate. Cut off from the compelling backstage workings of the barn, they simply lose interest once the novelty of wearing the snappy outfit begins wearing off. I can say this with confidence, not only because I've seen it happen, but also because I know that liking horses isn't really about money. It's about liking horses, and money helps.

But you can do horses on the cheap if you want to, and I am proof of that. After getting licensed to teach, I spent eighteen months as a working student and junior instructor at a forty-horse operation in Maryland, where I was paid twenty-five dollars a week to do the stalls, teach beginners, load hay, haul water, feed, clean tack, make repairs, and sweep the packed-clay aisle. My compensation package even included housing—a cold, dingy apartment over a garage where, when I unstoppered the bath, the tepid gray wastewater fell directly through the floor onto whatever unfortunate vehicle was parked below. The kitchen was dark, and the stove was spooky—if you turned any of the knobs it began to give off the hot, electrical odor of potential catastrophe. But I also rode in at least one private lesson a day, taught, worked the school and boarder horses, and sometimes had horses in supervised training. It was a glorious arrangement—I was busy, fit, and valuable, and it didn't cost a dime. Once it was over, I'd morphed into a reasonably competent horsewoman and, by my arithmetic, I was almost two hundred dollars ahead—this covered the cost of a plane ticket to my next barn, in South Carolina.

This kind of entry-level servitude is surprisingly common. Except for the top of the pyramid—the small number of winning racehorse owners, the double handful of Olympic-caliber trainers, riders, and support staff, and maybe a roomful of top dealers, teachers, and judges—most people who work in the horse business are just scraping along. It's not like the movie business, where even the lowliest crew member gets a salary and free sandwiches on the set, and it isn't at all like manufacturing furniture, where real profits are made, I suppose, from the need for whole societies to sit down somewhere other than on the floor. This is a difference not in degree, but in kind: The building of furniture is an obvious and useful industry and results in something made, something durable; even the motion-picture industry, for all its collateral fluffiness, has a definable product. The horse business is curiously intangible—if it's like anything, it's probably most like championship Scrabble or Civil War reenacting, driven by passion, not economics. It marches on, sucking up money by the bucketful, and it's not always clear, even to people in the thick of it, what's actually being accomplished. Yet the world of horses is a place of deeply felt imperatives—you can get in with money and you can get in with labor, but you can't stay in on any terms if the sight of a horse fails to move you.

This willingness to be moved by horses has several peculiarities, the most striking being that it shows up much more often in one gender. Girls and women are now the primary practitioners of the sport, and it's never been adequately explained why this is so. Vicki Hearne, writing in *Adam's Task*, touches briefly on this mystery when she observes that "Girls are . . . likely to become absorbed by the living allegory of horsemanship just at the age when their developing sexuality inspires the rhetorical forces around them to work harder than ever at distracting them from what they are interested in." Hearne's invocation of the word *interested* is more loaded than any ordinary usage, since she has just finished telling us about T. S. Eliot's observation about Blake, the poet, who "knew what interested him," and that this knowledge "made him terrifying." Blake is pretty terrifying, with his exclamation points and burning tigers, and Hearne points out that the faces of some older riders have a Blakean incandescence, a "gaze of unmediated awareness that one might be tempted to call innocence, since it is not unlike the gaze on the face of a child absorbed in Tinkertoys or a beautiful bug." But this expression comes at a price: "It is also terrible, the way Pasternak's face was terrible in its continuing steadiness of gaze."

This is interesting and perhaps truthful, but it skirts the question of why, when you go to the barn, you are mostly in the company of girls and women. An easy and uncomplicated explanation is that riding has something to do with sex—I've known any number of men who liked to make snickering references to saddles, the parts of my anatomy that saddles touch, and what all that might mean. The subtext was always that if I would just give up riding my horse, I could ride them, which would be better. The other explanation I've heard is that girls and women like to ride because it gives them power over something, and that women crave this power but must exercise it in some socially acceptable way. I'm the first to concede that many women have power issues—a fancy way of saying that we are almighty tired of being judged, poked at, and pushed around—but the real problem with the power argument is that, around the stable, exercising power for its own sake will never work. It is the horses who hold the cards and who must consent to the proceedings, and human powermongering invariably brings with it static, resistance, and bad results. Discipline matters, but it is the kind of discipline that is impartial and unrelenting, meted out pretty much equally on both sides. This makes riding one of those negotiated transactions where nobody really triumphs; if you are interested in scoring points off the animal, you will soon find yourself locked in a struggle you cannot control. If power is involved at all, it is of an unusually subtle, complex kind.

So this is a good question but a slippery one. Hearne, who writes about our lives with horses with depth and at times with intense accuracy, doesn't seem to know quite what to do with it, and resorts to the old literary trick of simply turning it inside out: "I have heard a number of people," she writes, "vaguely inspired by Freud, speculate about the passion for horses that develops in young girls. As a trainer, I came to see that the real question was not, 'Why do girls ride horses?' but rather 'Why don't boys?'"

But of course boys do, and even fill the top ranks of the sport in what seems to be slightly disproportionate numbers. There are various good reasons for this. Probably the most obvious one is that, until the period between the two world wars, most women still rode in a sidesaddle, and this is not a piece of equipment from which strenuous competition can be easily conducted. The sidesaddle, as a contraption, says a great deal about past societal attitudes toward women and horses, but none of it really bears repeating here; let us only clap and sing because those days are gone. But related to the sidesaddle was the plain fact that most competitive riding, at least in Europe, was very much a part of the military tradition. Since women were excluded from the ranks—and were riding sidesaddle to boot—it has taken time for them to get caught up. Especially in America, though, they've done a bang-up job of doing this—so much so that, in August 2000, I was actually caught a little off-guard by a wire report that appeared in the days leading up to Sydney Olympics. The headline read, "U.S. Show Jumping Team to Be an All-Female Affair," and what struck me at first was how silly this sounded. Would the same Associated Press journalist write a headline that went the other way, proclaiming that the U.S. team was exclusively male? This felt like gee-whiz reporting—the sportswriter, no doubt deeply accustomed to the widespread gender divisions in other sports, found novelty in something that didn't matter, since riding is one of the few endeavors where men and women compete as equals. But after my first reaction, the headline made me pause yet again, because it seemed to me entirely probable, even likely, that this really was the first time that the U.S. show-jumping team had been made up entirely of women. When you consider how thoroughly the lower and middle ranks are dominated by one gender, it's actually a little odd that women do not fill every slot when the Olympic team is selected.

But there is a final reason why men tend to be slightly overrepresented in the very top ranks, and it is because men are, by and large, bigger and stronger than women. Normally, size only matters in the sport in proportion to the horse you are sitting on—if your legs do not hang some critical distance down the sides of the animal, then you can't use them effectively. But because of the athletic demands of many of the phases of international competition, and especially the ones that involve large fences, long distances, strenuous movements, and time faults if you can't move along quickly enough, the top performance horses generally come in only two sizes—XL and XXL—in proportion to the questions being posed to them. And these big horses are, from a daily-contact point of view, not just large but also exasperating. The horror of a Grand Prix jumper is that he is a Grand Prix jumper, and he never lets you forget it; he is always singing his horsey, song-of-myself melody quite loudly in a high-pitched key. You want this sharp-edged personality during a high-stakes jump-off, but the time in between can be problematic—they are always *on*, like a high-powered lamp, always making announcements, always looking for something difficult and interesting to do. Men seem to enjoy a minor advantage in handling these wonderful but tiring creatures in that they tend to have more stamina. This isn't sexist; it happens to be true. This does not explain why there are so many girls and women who ride, but it probably does explain why there are more men in the very top tier of riders than would be dictated by probability.

But if you decide to look into this gender mystery, the necessary fieldwork can be downright baffling. When you listen to the young girls who hang around the barn, they often use charged, aesthetic, but surprisingly imprecise language to talk about the horses—they will tell you that Jimbo is a charmer, that Tinker is a real trouper, that Applesauce is a goofball or a big, sweet baby. It's hard to be sure what this kind of talk is meant to convey beyond affection, but it does tend to come across as anthropomorphic and trivial. Yet it is equally hard to take these young teens and preteens at their word, since there is a powerful disconnect between the way they coo and the way they actually interact with the horses: If you watch a junior rider, especially a skilled one, riding a horse she really understands, there is a sternness and a clarity there that is absorbing and impressive. Horse and rider may agree and disagree on various particulars, but the overall picture is one of shared commitment to getting something done, whether it be a change of lead at canter or a gymnastic combination of jumps. It's work, and you can see that it's work, but there is no air of drudgery about it; instead, the overwhelming impression is of interactivity and intense concentration. You don't need to know anything at all about riding to recognize this much, and you need to know only a little bit to feel that the spectacle is intrinsically beautiful.

This connectedness is a long way from effortless, but it is entirely the point. When riding teachers teach, they seem to work this metaphor harder than any other. One of my favorite ways of talking about it surfaced when Gina, one of the instructors at East Hill, said to a student, "Look, when you call somebody up on the telephone, you take turns, right? You don't just talk and talk and talk and then slam down the receiver. You wait. You want to see how your message got through; you need to find out what happened. You don't say the next thing until the last thing has been settled, and whatever you do, *you do not hang up the phone*."

Somewhere in this telephone metaphor is a concrete truth about girls and horses that may partially explain the gender phenomenon. Yes, horses are beautiful and lend status to their riders, but it isn't beauty or status that these girls are necessarily looking for. What they seem to need from their horses is a discussion—a *conversation*—with its flow of ideas, objections, proposals, counterproposals, rebellions, limits, reactions, and treaties. Conversations with horses are long-winded, probing, and fiercely individual, and the industry sometimes seems to be driven almost exclusively by girls and women searching for a horse who is interested in what they have to say.

FOUR

THE FIRST HORSE I LEARNED TO TALK TO WAS A HYPERACTIVE pinto mare. She'd initially been the property of my oldest foster sister, who, by the time I turned up in the family, had gone away to college and then graduate school. With accumulating age and lack of an interested rider, what had once been a big, fit, chocolate-and-white filly had become a slack-muscled, hairy, middle-aged mare, neurotic and a little sullen, more like an inmate than a domesticated animal. She was called Gem, a name that never fit her properly, and she spent the bulk of her time standing around in the stable yard looking like battered luggage in the wrong airport; her energy expenditures were hopelessly tangled up in tracking the whereabouts of her stable mate, a genteel bay Standardbred, and making a catastrophic racket whenever the two were separated. This second horse was regularly ridden, and because of this the mare had worn a deep track along the fence line, a kind of worry rut, from pacing and calling for her absent friend. This was the extent of her exercise. It wasn't much of a workout but she took it seriously, working up a whitish, worried sweat between her thighs. At the same time, she was a faded local legend—despite her current shabby presentation, she had been, in her younger days, a formidable jumper, and there were sun-bleached ribbons to prove it.

Jumping requires verve and speed, which Gem had in abundance, but it can also encourage the jitters, and it often takes a mental toll on any animal who is short on equilibrium to begin with, which Gem certainly was. She was talented, but her talent was embedded in her deficiencies, which began with distractibility and ended with high-stakes, hysterical resistance. This potent mix of athleticism and temperament was a problem for everyone who came in contact with her. She could *do* things, but whether she did them happily or willingly was a separate, difficult question. She'd been slightly pressure-cooked—not abused, and therefore not part of the mythology of the rogue—and the end result was that she assumed the things done to her by humans should be greeted with a fretfulness that was partly learned and partly genuine.

I didn't ride well, and she frightened me. My experience consisted of spotty but competent lessons and some ideas of my own picked up on borrowed animals. I could find my diagonals at the trot and my leads at the canter, but my rider's imagination was mostly filled with fuzzy ideas about what I can only call *correctness*—if you sat just so, and did things with the reins according to some protocol, then you were doing your part and things would be fine. It was mechanistic, but it was what I had. I didn't understand how fragile and even poverty-stricken this approach was; all I knew, especially at first, was that it wasn't working.

Just handling Gem with my feet on the ground gave me plenty to worry about—she was nearly uncatchable, and subterfuge was required to bring her up to be groomed and ridden. I learned to carry a roll of Necco wafers with me at all times—those thin, chalky candies that always struck me as refugees from the Depression era. Equipped with enough time and enough Necco wafers, I could catch her four outings out of five. But the overall arrangement was unsatisfactory—she didn't like being bribed and disliked herself, and me, for being party to such a dishonorable arrangement. Even I could see the resentment in her posture as she gave in to temptation and snatched the nasty candy. She pinned her ears as if to bite me and then pushed out a short, tense sigh.

Grooming was a drag, and we both hated it—she would not stand still. Some of this was her sensitive nature; she construed gentleness as tickling and almost everything else as painful, and the struggle to get her even passable—clean under the saddle and the future path of the girth—was an unpleasant ballet of dancing horse and defensive human. She stepped on me, hip-checked me against nearby objects, and swatted me with her big, hard skull. Her saving grace was that, for all her threats, she didn't actually bite or kick me, and after a while this began to stand out as an object of attention. Why didn't she? Even with my limited background, I knew that, with all the anger and anxiety in the air, kicking and biting should have been on the roster of possibilities. It took many months, but it finally dawned on me that this big mare was exasperating, spoiled, bored, quick to take offense, high energy, and probably as dumb as a box of rocks—yet despite everything that could be said about her, she wasn't mean. I hugged this tentative bit of knowledge. I was still afraid, but I found I was no longer particularly afraid of her. It was what might *happen* that scared me, and this is not the same thing.

Riding Gem was an intense, alert enterprise, in part because she had a very big go button but a tender mouth. She was rubbery and nimble and unusually easy to turn, but slowing her down took a lot of tact. The first few times I rode her, I reacted to her quickness with what seemed to me to be polite requests to take things at a more reasonable pace, and she immediately informed me that I had inflicted on her a powerful and painful insult. Several times during the first few weeks, she threw her head up so vigorously that it banged into my face; other times she would splay her front legs and jam them into the ground, stopping with a dramatic finality that sent shooting pains into my crotch and up my spine. She would freeze just long enough to feel my surprised hands release her and then bound forward again, forcing me to check her again; in this way we stopped, started, stopped, started, and thus jiggered our way miserably along the edges of the cornfields. It was a bit like riding a thousand-pound pogo stick.

Gem also startled easily, and was plagued by superstitions. She would go through periods of being deathly afraid of a certain red bucket, a tree stump, an article of my clothing. I learned not to wear the jacket with the hood; I forced her, for weeks, to eat a handful of grain out of the dreaded red horror; I got off and led her past the evil stump, cooing and comforting her the whole while. Soon enough I could wear the hood, leave the bucket in plain sight, and trot calmly enough past the offending amputated tree, but by then we had moved on to a horror of hoses, pie plates, and mailboxes. Things seemed to pop out of her environment, suddenly in high relief, and present a magnet for her huge quantities of free-floating anxiety; it was, as they sniggered on *Saturday Night Live*, always something.

Yet at the same time she showed invincible, impressive, unthinking courage. She would jump anything without adequate or prudent evaluation, she would gallop wildly down steep hills, she would cross narrow wooden bridges that swayed slightly under her considerable heft. Her belief in her own athleticism was unsettling but legitimate, since there seemed to be no real limit on what she could do, just limits on what I was willing to propose. She seemed to delight in my timidity, attacking physical challenges with a gusto that showered me with borrowed courage, but then something would distract her and she would begin bouncing, pulling, foaming, and waggling her ears. This mixture of anxiety and recklessness operated as an endless contradiction.

The only comfort I could offer myself about Gem was that I did not seem to be making things worse—she was horrid to everybody—but this reassurance was fragile, since I felt powerless to make things any better. Still, it was all I had, and I began to accept it. It sounds odd, but after the first year or so even her endless changeability was always the same, and I simply got accustomed to her shenanigans. This was not a good thing, but it was the easy thing, and if it weren't for my guilt and disgust over how we began every workout—the business with the Necco wafers—we probably would have gone on like that until the day she died or accidentally killed me.

Riding books—those tomes of *correctness*—never seem to address the things that really matter. They assume, falsely, that horses are interchangeable and that they offer up to their riders a generic and basically obedient equine personality. I suppose this is as it should be, since the goal of these books is to convey information about riding to riders, with the horse in a supporting role. But even books about dealing with problem horses do this; focusing almost exclusively on techniques humans can use to fix things; the bad horses in the books are cutouts, appearing only long enough to have their difficulties vaporized. Reading these books—and I read lots of them in my teens and early twenties—I knew there was something wrong about them but could not quite say what. They worked—sort of—in that I was following their advice about catching Gem, and I had to concede that I was, for the most part, catching her on an as-needed basis, but our shared misery was obvious. The books did not seem to think that this misery required any attention. Once the horse was caught, the problem was solved, and the text moved along to the next thing.

But I had also come to realize that what I hated most about catching my horse was the very thing that was recommended—

that resentful, resigned snatching of the Necco wafer. The wafer was inexpensive and got the job done, but it negated the whole point of the transaction. When horse and rider met, I had an idea that something interesting and good ought to happen, yet I was beginning all my encounters with Gem with a bait-and-switch operation that played only on her greed and her stupidity. I decided this was something I wanted to at least try to change. There was nothing to lose; if I failed, I could go back to the old system.

It was summer and both horses were out to grass, and the relatively wide-open spaces in the pasture were almost certainly going to work to my disadvantage, but I didn't want to wait. So I took up my lead rope and trekked to where Gem and her best friend grazed and swished at flies; they looked wonderfully peaceful. Then they both sensed me coming and their heads popped up—to this day I love this moment when horses acknowledge a new thing on their event horizon. It has a sharpness to it, a certain astringent acuity, that for some reason I find gratifying—it's both a reflex and a salute, those jack-in-the-box liftings of ears and eyes, the temporary high-beam watchfulness of seeking out the possible predator. Then they both made me, in the cop-show sense, and the loving and lovable Standardbred immediately began to pick her way toward me. Gem spied the lead rope and immediately began sifting away.

Ignoring Baby, as we all called the Standardbred—she had some registered name that was now nearly forgotten—I followed Gem. As soon as she sensed this, she picked up a little speed, jigging sadly into the upper reaches of the field where there was a small plantation of bushes she could use as impediments against me. She snaked her head and wrinkled her nose and made all the usual gestures that signaled her unwillingness to give in to being captured too easily. I watched while she settled into her protective mini jungle and then turned to keep a gimlet eye on me, and then

I did something I hadn't planned to do but now, feeling at a safe distance from the riding books stacked on my bedside table, was the first movement that occurred to me. I sat down.

The effect on Gem was immediate. She did another jack-in-the-box, alarmed by my sudden change in shape, and stared. Then her memory of the lead rope came back into play and she wrinkled her pink, slightly sunburned nose. I noted this and slid the rope underneath me, where for the next few paragraphs the metal snap dug quite hard into my fanny. Placated, Gem simply stood with her ears back and waited—she assumed that the ball was, as always, in my court, and her job was to react negatively to whatever happened next, which she assumed would be Necco wafers. As the minutes ticked by, a number of minor ideas seemed to occur to her, but apparently went nowhere. She couldn't resume eating, because the grass around the bushes was sparse and bitter; she couldn't leave, because that meant walking toward me, which was a violation of protocol; and she couldn't stand there forever, because, well, she couldn't. She tried chewing on the bush, but it was prickly and the experiment unsuccessful. She changed her position, castling herself the long way and the short way several times; she engaged in some prolonged and elaborate scratching and head rubbing, squashing her eyeballs noisily against her knees and sawing her nose against her cannon bone. Finally she just stood, thinking. This was hard for her but fascinating for me. For the first time since I'd met her, she was simultaneously alert, up to something, and perfectly still.

Finally Gem emerged from her citadel and stood in the open, obviously wondering what to do. My interest in her seemed a little unnerving—she wasn't used to scrutiny without interference—and for six steps she did the unthinkable and tiptoed toward me. Now it was my turn to worry—sitting on the ground when a large animal you know to be untrustworthy is approaching is not easy; I had a splendid view of her hard feet and an immediate awareness of her size. I felt sublimely kickable, but I reminded myself that she'd never deliberately hurt me. I also knew that what she was doing was hard for her, and it seemed only fair that I do something difficult in return. She stopped about eight feet away—too far for me to touch or catch her, but still very close by our understood standards—and looked down her nose at me. This nose seemed very big from the ground, and it gradually got bigger as she took another step and stretched to sniff me. Her whiskers dusted the top of my head. It was probably unnecessary, but she had confirmed my identity; I really was who I appeared to be.

I knew that, whatever happened, I must not try to catch her, so I did the next best thing—I gently shooed her away. I waved my hand quietly and said *git*, a voice signal that she had previously heard only at the end of being ridden, when I was done struggling with her and was putting her back in the yard or pasture. Despite its Western, twangy overtones, this signal doesn't really mean "run away," necessarily, so much as "you may now run away if you so choose"; it's a common locution used during routine horse handling, the rough equivalent of "all done" or "see ya." She knew what it meant, and I knew she knew, and its unsponsored appearance genuinely surprised her. She did *git* a little, stepping off a ways, but in less than a minute she was back within potential capture range. I said *git* again, and this time she decided to exercise her option to stay. After a little stalling and mulling things over, she dropped her head and showed me her halter: *Want some of this?* she seemed to say. The gesture was strangely flirtatious, as if she'd found herself in the possession of her own kind of Necco wafer. *Git*, I told her. *You are free to run away.*

But she wasn't free, and we both knew it, and it was time to bring the encounter to some kind of fruition. The next time she flirted with the halter, I conceded to touch it, but not where she anticipated. Instead of going for the snap ring under her chin, I reached up higher and undid the buckle on the side of her head so that the halter slid off her and landed in the dirt with a small metal-and-leather thud. Gem was amazed. Her ears pivoted in their sockets; if she'd been a cartoon horse, her eyes would have grown stems and steam would have come out of her ears. Now she *git* big time, tipping up on her toes and breaking off across the pasture, bucking and farting. She crashed happily into Baby, brimming with news. Baby flattened her ears and gave her a disciplinary punch with her closed teeth, then they gradually settled down to grazing again. Every few seconds, Gem shook her head mightily—not from the flies, but to confirm that her head was still unencumbered. She had a well-formed head, with high cheeks and a becoming nose, and I sometimes wonder if this was when I noticed its shapeliness for the first time.

FIVE

THE LANGUAGE OF REDEMPTION IS INCREDIBLY HARD TO manipulate, mostly because it has been co-opted by religion and the bottled-beverage industry. Yet it's important language, because redemption is one of the driving forces behind our talk both with and about horses—our stories about them are laden with ideas about value recaptured and an end to servitude, and these are both key meanings of the word. You can redeem another out of captivity or redeem yourself by making reparations for some bad action; these acts are both practical and moral, and the redemptive texts that operate in the world of horses are so pervasive that we sometimes fail to see that they are there. But they are. Monty Roberts, a trainer who is involved in the racing world and in Western riding, captures all these redemptive angles in his account of his life with horses.

Even in childhood, Roberts had an instinctive revulsion to the time-honored Western tradition of breaking horses to saddle by roping them, inducing panic, and keeping them panicked until they broke down mentally and became submissive. His horror of the process of sacking out—a burlap feed sack on a rope is used to incite terror in the untrained horse—is intensely felt and intensely moral. Watching his own horse being subjected to sacking out when Roberts was seven or perhaps eight years old was one of the turning points in his life. In *The Man Who Listens to Horses*, he wrote: "As I watched Brownie's eyes widen and roll in fear as he waited for what would happen next, I felt dread and sympathy. . . . I tried to think of how I might make it up to him, but I didn't know of a way." He does know the specific result of the trauma, however—by coincidence, Brownie was tormented not with the usual feed sack on a rope, but with a piece of heavy, crinkly paper originally used to line a crate of vegetables. "For his entire life," Roberts says, "he was phobic about paper. Anything that sounded like it would send him into a panic, and he'd be dangerous to himself and others. He would bolt madly, and no one could tell him that it was only paper, that it was nothing to be afraid of. I could never be angry with him for this blind spot in his nature and accepted it as our fault, our crime against him."

It probably doesn't matter very much that the vast majority of horses are introduced to being ridden with patience and careful handling, since what Roberts is really talking about is the widespread yearning among riders for rectification. This is certainly the predominant theme in horse stories; the genre, whether oral or written, is chock-full of horses just like Brownie, plagued by their human-made horrors. Anyone who has read these stories has probably grasped, intuitively, their moral and archetypal dimensions. Once the animal has rebelled and has thrashed, kicked, bit, stomped, or galloped his way into imminent peril, a child appears. This child acts as a shield between the horse and the adults who wish to punish or destroy the monster that they themselves have created; the child is also a rebuke and an emblem against the world's corruption. As has been noted by observers of the genre, the emotional and moral content of this kind of story is high, even pitched. Much is at stake, and the narrative requires that the threat to the horse be absolute: The bullet clicks in the chamber; cruel trainer unwinds his whip; the knacker's van pulls in the driveway. Or the danger can be less gory but still fraught: "In the hands of the right writer," Vicki Hearne points out, "the mere threat of being separated from the child is sufficient to make the horse's and the child's doom complete."

It's not enough that the child simply rescue the horse; the horse must also be transformed by the child, preferably into a mount who goes on to win widespread recognition for skill and virtue, and with these achievements comes the reversing of the destructive judgments made by various adults. Sometimes these adults merely change their minds about the horse; sometimes they are shamed by the horse's transformation in some public way; in extreme cases, the plot requires that all the mean grown-ups go to jail. Whatever happens, we can be sure it will be gratifying. The outcome is that the child and the horse are permanently linked. By saving the doomed animal, the child is also saved, and the world takes note of this transformation.

Horses cannot read and do not know these kinds of stories—if they did, then my problems with Gem would have melted away miraculously that summer morning when, instead of catching her, I set her free. We'll see that this is not how real horse stories really unfold, but that does not mean these stories are unimportant. They are, if for no other reason than they seem ubiquitous; we thrive on, and need, horse stories that are shamelessly redemptive. The underpinnings of these stories at first seem to insist that horses crave human understanding, and this is certainly an element in the storybook constellation, but the first principle of a good horse story is relief from abuse.

We have all heard stories about horses who were beaten and abused by a cruel trainer or handler, and this may be the single most common coin in the horse-narrative economy. For some reason—and perhaps it is some important reason—the abuser is almost always male. Over time, the horse is terrorized, not just by the presence of that individual, but by any individual who shares some salient characteristic. Trauma really does work this way, in that a horrible memory is easily triggered by some detail—a gesture, the smell of a certain type of cigar, a porkpie hat—and, once triggered, it plays itself out in an escalating badness that is thinly disguised panic. Like Brownie's reaction to the rustle of paper, there are cues, however small, that can rob a horse of his mental equilibrium. These stories are very widespread, and a certain proportion of them are undoubtedly true.

That said, though, I would like to raise a few questions about these abused-horse stories as a whole class of narrative, since there really are some obvious problems. First, they are amazingly common: It seems you can't talk to ten owners without encountering at least five who tell you their horse was beaten and abused at some time in the past. "You just can't wave your hands near his face at all," you're told, "because he was beaten over the head." But the plain truth is that no horse likes having things waved near his face; an objection to flapping is a normal response, and we do not need a story to justify it. The second problem with these stories is that you often hear them from riders who are failing on some level with their animals—they sometimes turn up at clinics, where they waste everybody's time because of their horse's disruptive behavior, or at competitions, where their mount pulverizes every fence or refuses to enter the arena at all. When the stewards approach or the clinic instructor asks if the rider would please be excused, the abused-horse story is invoked as a way of casting the trainer or rider in a heroic role.

Without discounting every instance of the abused-horse story—I have an idea that perhaps one in eight may actually be true—it's easy to see that these are fraudulent uses of what is obviously a resonant, useful narrative. But it needs examining mostly because it is so resonant, and because its momentum is derived from a real, really horrible truth that we can barely face: All riders, however accomplished they may be right now, have behaved badly toward some horse at some time in the past. There are no exceptions to this dreary rule. The bad treatment may have been done out of ignorance, inexperience, or frustration, but there is no rider who can escape the charge of cruelty. Good intentions do not count; all people who like horses live with the shame of knowing a horse who does not like them in return, and many skilled riders have a damaged horse not only on their conscience but in their barns. This is the kernel of truth that the abused-horse story forms around, acquiring layers of meaning and drama, and in some important way it acts as the first chapter of the classic horse story, but one that is still waiting for the happy ending. Otherwise, to accommodate all the abused horses we hear about, we'd almost need a factory somewhere, running several shifts, where minimum-wage sadists systematically ruin animals as a final step before putting them on the market.

But abused-horse stories need not be true to be truthful, and it's worth noting one last thing about them: To be really useful, they must be outgrown. Maybe it's a developmental thing, like pivot grammar in toddlers, but the whole class of narrative at some point has to be abandoned before a rider can cross a Rubicon into the land where responsible riding actually unfolds. All trainers acknowledge that horses are imperfect and come with their fair share of problems, and the best trainers accept that horses often arrive draped in melodramatic stories that may or may not be worth listening to. As we'll see later, at least one person in this book understood the importance of not hearing a horse's story before beginning the hard work of redemption. This is exactly as it should be: Horses live in, and genuinely prefer, the present tense, and their mental bandwidth is far more likely to be used up by a bright square of unexpected sunlight on the dark floor of an indoor arena than by mulling over indignities, however harsh, inflicted two years or even two weeks ago. It is not that horses do not tell themselves stories—I think they do—but that their stories are not human and not particularly accessible. Humans talk about rectification and time; horses, it seems, talk mostly about tigers and space.

Research and observation have shown that horses have complicated and even byzantine thoughts about space. Like most animals, including humans, they have ideas about their personal space—the area immediately around them that is rightfully theirs—and also carry around with them a wider spatial bubble that they use for managing threats. This larger zone is sometimes called a flight distance, and it tends to extend a long way behind most horses but not particularly far in front of them—a startled mare will almost always escape to the far edge of her flight bubble before turning around to take a look at whatever tiger might be coming after her. Horses, as a species, believe firmly in tigers, even though domesticated horses rarely encounter them; this is not stupid but adaptive. Horses are edible and relatively defenseless, and much of their evolutionary history has been all about not being eaten, and most of the things that want to eat them come up stealthily from behind. This explains why, if you want to catch a wily mare in an open field, it is best to loop around and approach her from the front, where the flight distance is small and there is more opportunity for an exchange of signals and other forms of negotiation before she has to make a decision about what she is going to do. People who don't understand this can spend huge amounts of time trekking sadly behind a horse who just keeps going indefinitely—and she *will* keep going indefinitely, or at least for as long as the human keeps acting like a tiger.

There's nothing particularly remarkable about this understanding of space—it's a fairly off-the-rack herd-animal response—but it exasperates novice handlers because it seems to make no sense. Humans, after all, behave differently: We tend, as a species, to go *toward* novelty, movements, and noises in the underbrush, mostly because our predatory curiosity trumps the possibility of tigers. From our human perspective, the behavior of the horse seems stupid and intransigent, and may seem stupider still when, after an hour or so of trudging, we give up the pursuit and decide to head back to the house for dinner. Then the dynamic often reverses itself so that the horse we have been following is now following us. This happens with some regularity because all horses are generically tempted by following—it's another powerful and adaptive herd impulse—and the elusive mare may even catch up and follow us fairly closely, now that we are no longer acting like a tiger, and allow herself to be caught. Many handlers who report these encounters think they are being teased by the animal, but the real cause is buried in the fairly complex way that horses interpret and manipulate space.

Horses also seem to carry with them very distinct ideas about the shape, uses, and dimensions of the world. Left to their own devices outdoors, a group of horses will settle into a home range and then select out the places in it where they will loaf, roll, play, eat, poop, and socialize, and all this is done without any reinforcement or even particular notice from their human handlers. Many horses even carry this desire to organize space back into the stable and apply it to their box stalls, where they develop rituals about eating, dunging, snoozing, and carrying out their various indoor vices like cribbing, wind sucking, and weaving. In the same vein, horses can also develop places in the riding arena that are sweet spots, where they feel forward and chipper, or ugly ones, where they are more likely to balk and snivel.

In short, horses are *mappers*. Anyone who has ridden out on trails or in open country on a horse has almost certainly noticed the unassailable competence they enjoy not just in being able to always get home again, but in being able to do it even in strange country. Lucy Rees, in *The Horse's Mind*, says,

> Allowing a horse to "home" from a place he has not been before is a fascinating exercise, for it allows us to appreciate what cues are important to a horse in his normal wanderings. When turning back after a long ride into strange country they often use smells at junctions of paths, sniffing each one intently before setting off briskly on the right one. . . . When they take a "wrong" path it usually turns out to be a short cut back to the right one, though whether they are using landmarks or a sense of direction is not known. Whatever they are using, they are better at homing than we are, as many a lost or tired huntsman or horseman has had good reason to appreciate.

Rees conveys, without actively saying, that horses perk up when offered the opportunity to find their way home through new territory, and this is generally true. Horses share with humans the joy of doing something interesting that they are good at, and mapping is one of the great strengths of the equine intelligence. Horses remember and map where bad things happened—a talent they are often punished for—and also where delightful things once occurred. Thus a horse who once met a tiger (or perhaps it was a rabbit) on the edge of a certain field will always be in a heightened state when he approaches the edge of that field again, and if his heightened state makes his rider nervous, he usually decides that there is well and truly something serious to worry about there. If the rider starts notching her way up the anxiety scale and becomes actively afraid, then so does the horse—it simply does not occur to him that the rider might be afraid of *him*, only that the rider can see yet another, perhaps larger tiger, hidden from his equine view. This can have a snowball effect, and all sorts of further mapping can easily follow, most of it unproductive. The fault lies not in the horse, necessarily, or even in the rider, but in the murky space between them that is full of the different things they do and do not know.

This gap between horse and rider is sometimes full of misunderstanding, but it can be crossed with the right kind of conversation. Gem was proof of that. After my encounter with her in the pasture, which I repeated over a few days with some minor variations, Gem began to get actively involved in what we were doing. On the face of it, it did not seem like we were doing very much—I would go out, fool with her halter, change my shape, catch her, release her, proclaim her goodness, and then go away again—but she soon began walking toward me across the grass, cautious but alert, invested in the next installment of this interesting game. I was happy because I was getting something I really wanted, since we now began each encounter on a good note; I saw that she was happy, or at least engaged, by a string of encounters that were painless and new. It seemed to me an arrangement worth preserving, and for a couple of weeks I cut back on riding her while we spent a lot of time just messing around together in the pasture. I began putting her on a longe line (this is pronounced *lunge*, and is just a French way of saying "long") and asking her to wobble around at the end of it. I had seen other people longe their horses, and it didn't look all that hard. The longer stood more or less in one place; the longee went around in a circle. Gem seemed to know something about it, which was a relief, since it gave me less explaining to do, and I quickly learned a great deal about her because I could actually see her, something that is impossible to do on board.

I knew from riding her that Gem had a flexible, almost slinky quality—she moved more like a huge beagle than with the clock-work cadence of a regular horse—but that this rubbery lightness was fragile and could be interrupted by attacks of the herky-jerkies that, particularly when I longed her, always seemed to happen whenever my own attention began to wander. All I had to do to get her pogo-sticking and stomping around was to glance at a passing car, the ground, or the longe line in my hands, which through inexperience was often a disorganized tangle. If I paused to pick at a knot, she jiggered; if I still insisted that the longe line was more important than she was, she would buck or bolt. It took me a while, but I figured out that if I wanted her to be good, or at least not disruptive, I had to pay real attention to her and actively hold her in my gaze. This surprised me, since I had come to think that she was more or less indifferent to me—if I mattered to her at all, it was because I irritated and interfered. Yet here was something she really wanted, and for once it was something I could give. As I got the knack of handling the equipment—forty-odd feet of line and an utterly harmless lightweight whip—I bungled less and gave her more of my undivided attention.

The immediate effect of this attention was that her posture and manner on the circle became not only more consistent but more intense. She wanted me to see her, to watch her feet, to no-tice her big round fanny, to admire the slope of her shoulder. I thought I was imagining this, but the idea would not go away—it was so persistent that I even began to wonder if she knew *where* I was looking. If I looked at her head, she tended to tuck her chin and move more smartly; if I looked at her barrel, she twitched her skin, ridding herself of imaginary flies. If I dropped my eyes down to her feet or back to her hindquarters, she slowed down noticeably. This was fairly weird. In all the riding books I'd read, none had ever indicated that the beam of a handler's eye could be actively felt and responded to, and for a while I simply failed to believe it was really happening, even though it was.

But there was also a global change. It seemed that Gem actually expanded with all this looking, growing and widening before me, enjoying what was clearly for her an oblique, subtle touching. I had an idea that, on some level, this was the only kind of grooming she could stand. With practice, I could even get her to change direction using only gestures and changes in my own posture and position: Gem would brake, pivot handily, and be miraculously reversed and back on her rubbery way. There was an obvious element of play in the way she executed this movement, as if we were having a game of tag, and as she moved off in the new direction her expression can only be described as thoughtful and perfectly satisfied. After about a week, as we got better at aligning our cues, she absentmindedly volunteered a few slow, rounded steps of canter, executed with an absence of fuss that was utterly untypical of her. I was impressed, and she could tell.

I am sorry to report that this new horse I was handling in the pasture was speedily replaced by the old horse as soon as I got on her again—horses stubbornly refuse to play along with our ideas about redemption. But there was something about this series of encounters that I found pleasantly mysterious, as if I had been offered a tantalizing one-word clue or perhaps half a map with part of an X on it. We went back to the jigging and the bursts of speed and the imaginary dangers (bicycles! garage doors! bird feeders!), but my new way of catching her and our pasture play somehow held against the tide of her excitability. She now came to me quietly, and with an air of inquiry, and I understood that this involved more than just a change in my technique. The marginal temptation of the Necco wafer had somehow morphed into a temptation with *me*. I was, at least some of the time, a provisional partner in the Gem enterprise.

SIX

THE DAYS STAYED COLD UP AT EAST HILL BUT THEY WERE AT least starting to get longer, and the improved authority of the sun sometimes meant that there were actual puddles in front of the main barn door when I arrived for my lesson. The air began to smell yeasty—a sure sign that the season was really going to change—and an exposed section of the driveway was sometimes squishy or had refrozen into deep ruts that grabbed the car and heaved it in unexpected directions. Mud is the first sign of spring in Vermont.

As the season and the lessons began to progress, I dug through a box at home and discovered a couple of pairs of riding breeches I'd worn while competing in college. I was triumphant to find that they still fit, sort of, although my boots did not. I'd taken up lap swimming in my forties, and my legs had become thicker and harder as a result, so when I hooked my old black dress boots to my boot pulls I had to puff and lean for a good fifteen minutes. They finally slid on, but then immediately began to hurt; this pounding, congested pain was soon followed by another bout of puffing and pulling so prolonged that I began to worry I would never get them off again.

I wanted to dress better than my usual chaps, jeans, and hiking boots because the situation was starting to demand it, not just because the riding was getting strenuous but because of Prince. Prince enjoyed his work, and understood it, and there was something about his composure and reliability that made me want to honor him. His temperament made my lessons with him infinitely easier: I was in some sense superfluous to his larger mission, but he invariably absorbed my clumsy attempts to do dressage on him with an impenetrable good humor that seemed to come from the core of his princely being. We circled, flexed, fumbled, and dribbled, and never once did Prince show any temper. On the contrary, he was always delighted to see me (he liked the grooming), and each time I put my clumsy self aboard, my long leg swinging over his short back and settling against his side, he absorbed me with a spongy willingness—I was just another mess that Prince had been assigned to clean up. He then set forth into a sea of trouble—static, mixed messages, and rider confusion—without comment or resentment. It seemed the least I could do from my end was put on some presentable clothes.

The first thing I needed to get squared away was a new kind of steering. All my life I had turned horses with my hands, relying on my legs and my seat as backup mechanisms, and it had never crossed my mind that this might not be the best way to get the turning job done. If I wanted to go left, I would pull on the left rein, using my left hand either as an opening rein or as a simple direct rein; on a more experienced horse, I sometimes also used an indirect rein, a sort of pushing rein on the neck using the hand away from the turn. Whatever I did, however, involved pressure of some description. These make-a-turn techniques were deeply ingrained in my neural system, no doubt because they had the advantage of really working. Horses turned, and to date no horse had complained, and these good results meant I didn't think about it. There are so many other things that hands have to accomplish while riding—contact, straightness, speed, general control of the situation—that the whole cornering thing seemed to be a minor detail.

The wrongness of this basic protocol amazed me. Turns, I learned from Prince, had nothing to do with hands. When I turned Prince in my regular way, he merely bulged, turning his head and neck to indicate he heard me but choosing his own line of travel. Navigation became approximate—we would noodle around on the diagonal line across the arena, heading for the far corner marker, and about half the time we never even arrived there, or arrived in a state of befuddlement, his haunches swinging like a car on new black ice. Circles were lopsided eggs, and each egg had its small end in some different part of the arena. Kathie had a whole set of language that addressed this—Prince was "escaping," "avoiding," and "going on two tracks," and she told me, over and over and in different ways, to stop relying on my hands and fingers. But what else was I to rely on? That part wasn't clear.

Then, one cold March day, we did a strange exercise. I was told I was now going to stop Prince without using my hands at all. Say what? Kathie insisted that it could be done. Like turning, this seemed to me an utter contradiction, but Kathie had already been proved right on several fronts that seemed inexplicable to me, so I settled down to listen. "You walk, and you move your seat, right? You let yourself follow his movement. So now all I want you to do is stop following his movement. You're not really resisting, you're just not following. And your hands close around the rein. Not pulling. They just close, and wait for him. And when he gets there, you hold for a moment and then release."

This sounded pretty stupid to me, but I could see that Kathie was a true believer, so we dribbled out onto the rail at a walk on a fairly short rein. "Shut your eyes," she said. Prince was utterly trustworthy, so I did. In the stringy-dotted darkness behind my eyelids, I could feel the bouncy cadence of Prince's walk.

"Listen," Kathie said.

"Do what I say.

"You are walking.

"Follow his back, follow his back, follow his back.

"Now don't follow. Stop your seat and close your fingers.

"Now relax them.

"See?"

I did see, mostly because I cheated and opened my eyes. In the mirror on the long wall I could see that Prince had squared himself up into a sweet, obedient halt, one ear cocked at Kathie and, for the first time, one ear actually cocked back toward me.

Riding is not a sport heavily laden with *aha* moments—it's not theoretical physics—but I knew that something significant had happened. It wasn't just the bizarre mechanics of the thing, but the sensation that accompanied it: For the first time I felt the sprightly pegs of Prince's hind legs as a living presence under me, and the beam of his attention. We halted several times in this new way, and it was great fun. Each time I managed it successfully, suppressing my desire to merely pull, I felt something old and familiar: Prince seemed *magnified*. Like Gem on the longe, Prince grew and became a larger presence under me, emanating his pony pleasure in the world, and after the third good halt he dropped his head, met my hands with his narrow jaw, and chewed. "*Now* he's thinking about coming into the bridle," Kathie said. "Can you feel that?"

"Room," I replied. "Some poo."

"I'll take that as a yes."

If you can stop a horse without pulling, then it follows that you can also turn. It's harder, and it's probably not wise to shut your eyes, but at least I had a vestigial feeling for what might be involved. The turn, it seemed, no longer originated from things in front of me—my hands, his mouth—but from something under me and behind me, from the touch of his hind leg on the springy footing of the arena. It could be accomplished by thoughts about turning, and by making turns originate in the wet innards of my body; at least part of the time now, we produced round, effortless circles that seemed to have their beginnings in a corner of my lower back and a tiny signal emanating from my hip. And once I could turn Prince in this new way, I discovered that he immediately assigned me much more credibility. For the first time, he began to get a little grumpy when I rode him in the old, front-ended way, which Kathie called "push–pull" riding. Prince was unwilling to be a push–pull horse, and when I resorted to pushing and pulling he behaved as if I had failed to meet some basic standard or, more accurately, that I was guilty of backsliding. Prince now expected something specific from me, and would tolerate nothing else, and I basked in the weight and purity of this demand.

Horses will sometimes make these unilateral policy changes in their relations with humans, despite a general insistence, in riding literature, that this is not the case. Henry Wynmalen, in his *Dressage: A Study of the Finer Points of Riding*, says it most clearly: "The main thing to remember is that it is the trainer who makes the horse; it is he and he alone who is responsible for good and bad results alike." Wynmalen is among the least obscure and most charming of the writers who try to wrestle riding into prose, and his love of the species pokes through everywhere, but on this matter he takes the conventional position: Riders are responsible for all results. Yet they aren't, not always. At least some of the horses I have known have accepted and even insisted on their own specific contribution, their own responsibility. Even setting Gem aside, and Prince, I once had a horse in a school string named Camouflage who steadfastly refused to comply with any rider's bad idea, whether that be approaching an obstacle from a foolish angle or breaking into a canter before the rider was ready. All riding teachers eventually encounter a horse or two like this, and acknowledge, at least to themselves, that these creatures have an independent integrity, a kind of proactive equilibrium that they use to maintain order and safety inside the frame that horses care about. It is no good arguing that these horses are beautifully trained, since most are only adequately schooled at a fairly low level, and yet they somehow bring to the lesson far more than their own lessons ever brought to them. Cammie, as we called this Appaloosa gelding, was not a particularly pleasant or accommodating personality—he went at his work with a vengeance, and this made him humorless—but he was irreplaceable.

In light of these kinds of equine transactions, it's worth wondering—how much do horses really understand? The answer, always, is that it depends on the horse, but at East Hill all the horses seem to understand the ebb and flow of activity, the nuances of the feeding routine, the turnout schedule, and the schooling-and-lesson roster, and some of the horses may even have makeshift ideas about time that correspond roughly to our days of the week. This is human knowledge, in the sense that they learn it from us and use it to make sense of our behavior, and our judgment of whether a horse is good, less good, or even evil is at least partly keyed to a horse's ability to observe and comply with the codes of conduct that operate in individual barns.

But horses also know many other things that have nothing to do with us, just as humans know many things—theoretical physics, say—that have nothing to do with them. Horses are very interested in sniffing things, for example, particularly the urine and feces of other horses; most humans find this puzzling, distasteful, and something to be discouraged. At East Hill, there is a large rubber bucket placed near the cross ties so that, when a horse defecates while being groomed or tacked up to be ridden, the rider can clean up quickly and easily. These droppings accumulate in the bucket and are of general interest to every passing inhabitant, especially if they are fresh and still steaming. The horses, and particularly the geldings, can be wholeheartedly insistent about plunging their faces into the muck bucket, and seem to greet fresh dung as a form of aromatherapy. It's pretty gross.

But what's gross to us is urgent for them, since sniffing dung is a social exercise. When you ride out across the countryside and encounter a horse-dung pile, any horse with a proper interest in life will want to give it a good going-over. From this sniffing, horses seem to gather intelligence about the gender and perhaps even the age and physical status of the responsible party, although it's hard for us humans to say, exactly, what else they learn and why it's important. But it *is* important—horses are intensely social beings, and one of the sad by-products of being handled by humans is that we tend to subvert their desire to clump together, form and sustain complicated relationships, conduct friendships, hold grudges, and generally carry on a rich emotional life, of which dung sniffing is a component. Certainly one of the things that horses know, unequivocally, is that living outdoors in a group is better than standing alone in a box stall, and it is a credit to the species that they consent to it at all.

Horses also know that different human beings are really different. This doesn't sound like much of an achievement, since we humans can tell each other apart so easily, but many humans are sorely challenged to tell one horse from another. I can, but only because I've had some practice; it's an acquired skill. Most movie directors don't have it, and they sometimes use horses in their films as if they were interchangeable. Thus the same chestnut mare with the high white socks appears in one scene carrying a Lakota brave and in the next as an equine member of the U.S. Cavalry, and in both takes she offers the viewer the same markings, head shake, expression, and posture, and shows the same distinctive, hopping transition into canter. This obvious inconsistency is annoying to people like me, who take note of the horses, but it mostly proves my point: Directors carefully reset clocks and manipulate sets, lights, objects, and clothing to achieve what is called cinematic continuity, but errors like this are utterly invisible to them, and probably to the majority of moviegoers. In general, people are much less observant about horses than horses are about people.

Horses track individual humans by our smells, our gestures, our crimes, and our acts of comfort and clarification, and it does not take many encounters for a horse to lay down a recognition track for a specific individual. If the encounter is even vaguely memorable, it only takes one. Prince, for example, clearly knew me the second time I met him, since he perked up noticeably as I approached with my brushes and attempted, right off the bat, to groom me in return. This mouthy, damp attention is not something humans generally welcome—it's easy to interpret having your shoulder nibbled as an act of aggression, even though it's meant to be sociable. Plus it only hurts a little, but this is not the point. The point is that even school horses, who are ridden and handled by hundreds of different people over a lifetime, seem to sort out quickly who is who and act accordingly, although it must be added that many school horses—including the good ones like Camouflage—develop withdrawn, stoic, and defensive personalities. Otherwise the chaos of coping with so many different riders might well drive them crazy. But even among that tolerant tribe, there are degrees of responsiveness that are clearly based on individual recognition. Prince, as I learned later by watching him in the fields, is an unusually extroverted personality—he forms powerful attachments to other horses and initiates a lot of hobnobbing—and this strong social drive pops out, with very little coaxing, in his relationships with people.

Horses know us with an intimacy and a limited, laserlike accuracy that can be truly disconcerting, and it's hard to be sure how or why this has happened. The transfer of social interest from a member of your own species to a creature with a different outline, agenda, and form of locomotion is a strange achievement, and it is an achievement specific to domesticated animals. Dogs clearly have it, and cats, despite their postures of denial and misdirection, have it, too; it could be that individual wild animals can acquire it, although hand-fed, supposedly tame raccoons often remain permanently problematic. I understand that they like to play, but I also understand that they like to bite, escape, and wreck things. They do not really manifest the essential prerequisites of domestication: the willingness to join the human enterprise in exchange for room, board, paid medical, and job security. It's not that wild animals can't be fed by hand—they can—but they do not understand the contract. They belong to themselves; truly domesticated animals seem to accept that we belong to each other.

Yet horses, as one of the East Hill blacksmiths reminds me, are not really pets. He does this, perversely, by saying that they are. I am hanging around and watching him work on a refined, rather edgy black mare named Tutte, who has recently gone mysteriously lame. Tutte stands in the cross ties and conveys all sorts of messages about having her feet worked on—she wriggles and sometimes even flinches as the nails go in—while the owner and the blacksmith talk about her recent soundness problem. The vet, who has looked at her, has suggested that her shoes should be

pulled and her feet inspected, but the blacksmith has found nothing—no abscess, no bruising, no cracking, no punctures, no signs
of injury. Tutte's feet look basically fine.

Tutte, however, is not fine, and her ongoing, worried protest
makes the blacksmith yearn out loud for the olden days. He steps
back and watches her fidget for a moment, and then says, "You
know, when horses had real work, farm work, they didn't make such
a dumb fuss about things like this. You all think you make them
work, but you really don't. Look at her. She's nothing but a pet."

To my surprise, the owner agrees. "You're right," she says.
"You know, a few years ago I told my husband that I had to have
either another baby, an affair, or a horse. He knew I really meant
it, so we figured it out. Kids are expensive, and for some reason he
didn't like the idea of an affair. That left the horse."

This is meant to be funny and self-deprecating. This particular owner—a retired teacher with a raffish, glinting, talkative
charm—sometimes agrees with people just to keep a happy conversation going. But Tutte, nodding and shifting and swishing her
tail, does not seem very petlike; she seems sore and preoccupied.
Driving home from the barn, I think about this exchange, wondering why it bothers me so much, and finally realize that the word *pet*
is problematic when applied to a horse. It seems to me that pets, as
a class of beings, really have to be smaller than us. This rule has
something to do with the word itself; *petting* a horse is a pointless activity, unrelated to the horse's genuine function, and is understood
by some horses as a form of teasing. You sometimes pat a horse on
the shoulder and give him a word of praise, but this is a signal; if
you want gratifying hand-to-skin contact with a horse, you groom
him, which is goal-directed and, as I've tried to convey, surprisingly
complicated. Petting, at least with horses, is at once trivial and condescending, in that the animal is expected to be grateful, whether
he is or not; petting for its own sake is done to gratify the humans,

and seems to come up most often in the form of a request from couples with small children: "Can my little girl pet your horse?"

But even if we set aside the objections to the word *pet*, it's also clear that horses are not really *companion animals*, either—this is probably just a politically correct *pet* upgrade, but it does have the advantage of describing, in a nontrivial way, what some domestic animals, most often dogs, are really doing. Yet horses *don't* do it—horses do not curl up at the foot of the bed, and perhaps more importantly they do not want to; like cattle and other claustrophobic barnyard animals, they much prefer the outdoors. Nor do horses want to come along on your errands, protect your interests, evaluate your houseguests, or guard your property. But on the other hand a horse is also not like a cow, even though cows are also clearly domesticated. I have met many cows and worked briefly with some of them, and it's clear that, despite thousands of years of selective breeding, cows are not really very interested in humans. They seem to see us as appliances, dispensing nutrition and removing excess fluids, an attitude that leaves them free to be cows. There's nothing wrong with this—far be it from me to criticize so useful a creature—but our relations with cows tend to be morally undifferentiated. By this I mean that, even though it's easy enough to tell one cow from another with contact and practice, as far as I know we do not tell heroic stories about cows, or describe them with language like *honest, trappy,* or *educated.* That we use these words with horses, and use them all the time, does not mean we have fallen down the rabbit hole of anthropomorphic thinking. What it means, I think, is that the blacksmith is mistaken.

One of the chronically exasperating things about our species is that we tend to think that the only notable thing about animals is that they are not human. They are animals, and that is somehow enough—people say they "like animals" or are "good with ani-mals," as if all animals are the same. Yet the difference between a blue jay and a hedgehog is substantial, and the difference between the blue jay and the hedgehog is a different kind of difference than the one between a Great Dane and a giraffe. Yet we, as a species, mostly act like cows, in that we do not differentiate—we even have a cable TV channel, Animal Planet, where the pro-gramming seems to consist almost exclusively of home video footage shot relentlessly from this bovine point of view. The squir-rel stuck in the bird feeder is put on the same condescending and comic footing as the cockatoo wearing roller skates, which is equiv-alent to the puppy who pulls down the toddler's pants, exposing a charming pink behind. This cascade of imagery never seems to pause, even for a moment, to remind us that the puppy is teething, the wild squirrel is in trouble, and the cockatoo—well, let's not go there. Let's just say it's a depressing spectacle.

I am not good with this undifferentiated mass of beings called "animals," although I've been told by lots of people that I am. I suspect that this is mostly because I don't approach dogs whom I don't know as if I had a constitutional right to invade their privacy, and one result of this is that most dogs don't worry much about me. This does not qualify as being "good with animals"; all it really means is that I don't get snubbed or bitten. This is not a virtue, and only exists because I am shooting much, much lower: I would like, someday, to be good with one and perhaps as many as three horses. Maybe I'll get there; in the meantime, I am frankly mysti-fied by my cat, Petunia, who has lived with me for seventeen years and who will still not swallow a pill and who seems to enjoy cast-ing me in the role of her oppressor. I get bogged down in struggles with her that I do not understand, mostly having to do with spatial matters—how furniture ought to be used and arranged, the de-ployment of litter boxes, and the precise angle that a door should be held open before she will consent to pass through it. Many of the things that are urgent for Petunia seem to me a complete waste of time; she, in turn, disapproves of my obsession with the computer keyboard and walks across it disparagingly whenever she can. Much of her time is spent doing surveillance—she notes my comings and going with obvious consternation, like a supervisor with an unsatisfactory worker—and these observation periods are punctuated by sporadic explosions of rug shredding, pencil rolling, and plaintive commentary. She will sometimes lie on my chest, purring loudly and drooling, but she only initiates these love fests when I am freshly home from work and stretched out to read the mail; she almost certainly knows my routine well enough to anticipate that within moments I will get up off the sofa to start cooking dinner. Thus the disruption she herself has manufactured becomes grounds for further insult. Weirdly, she does not treat anyone else this way. Her relations with other members of the household seem perfectly neutral and pleasant—I am the exclusive object of her note taking and her beady gaze, and the subject of whatever lengthy petition she is secretly composing. This is obviously a very complicated relationship, but it's one that only Petunia understands. Does this sound like "good with animals" to you?

My point—and I seem to have gone far afield to reach it—is that some horses may exhibit petlike and even pettish behavior in that they may seem stuck or fussy or excessively sensitive, but it comes from a different source. The horse–human entanglement has plenty of room inside it for ruination and misunderstanding, but a fussy horse and a fussy cat are as different from each other as they are different from a fussy child. When put in these terms—and especially when you put the human in there (as if we were also animals, which we are)—the business of judging the status of the fuss becomes much more challenging. Still, it is worth the work. Once you acknowledge that different species are genuinely different, it becomes possible to do what many horses do so well, which is to calibrate other creatures as individuals.

As for Tutte, who was last seen flinching rather girlishly in the cross ties, it fell out that she had a hairline fracture of the coffin bone, a weight-bearing yet strangely porous bone in the foot. I once had the opportunity to hold a coffin bone, and it feels like a sculpted bit of pumice; in a living horse, these holes and fissures are packed with blood vessels that feed the horn of the hoof. A fracture in this surprisingly delicate structure is going to hurt, and pounding nails into the hoof wall—normally a painless proce-dure—is going to make it hurt even more. Some surgical shoeing and a long period of rest will probably put her right. Still, her fuss was justified, and I bring this diagnosis up mostly to remove any lingering stain on Tutte's character.

SEVEN

ADULT WEEK AT EAST HILL IS HELD EVERY APRIL AND IS A chance for the gainfully employed middle-aged women who ride there to take time off from work and focus on horses. There are seven of us. The agenda is simple and summer-campy: We ride, help with barn chores, and attend various riding and management demonstrations during the day, while in the evening we all converge at Con and Jeanette's house, which is next to the barn and overlooks the outdoor dressage arena. There we watch horse videos, eat raw vegetables with dip, and drink the kind of wine that comes in those big boxes with a little spigot at the bottom. These videos are frequently paused so we can talk about what we see. Then we have a group dinner at Jeanette and Con's large oval dining table—the various barn staff take turns preparing something—and by the time the evening is over, we are all pleasantly worn out, full, and ready for tomorrow, when it all happens again. It's meant to be fun, and it is, but it's also serious: Riding skills improve dramatically when you get instruction every day. To my surprise, Adult Week isn't particularly expensive—just a little more than the cost of five regular lessons in a row.

The videos we watch often have us in the starring roles, since we tape each other's lessons, then sit in a tense row on the couch and on the floor and watch them with a kind of fascinated horror. All of us know at least something about getting around on a horse, or thought we did, but the images on the screen seem to prove otherwise: "What *is* that with my hands?" Katherine wonders; "If I'm going to bounce like that, I need a better bra," says Cindy; "Oh God Oh God Oh God," says Judy. I decide to stick with an embarrassed silence. There is tiny Prince, looking cockeyed and ebullient, tromping around among the normal-sized horses with his ears twirling and his thick tail bouncing in a repeating and graceful *S*, but he is burdened with a giant slob who seems bent on interference and once, to my infinite shame, catches him in the mouth as he steps into canter. It's disgraceful; I've never really seen myself ride before and had no idea I am so utterly without finesse. Worse, I had done a little jumping that day, just to take a break from nonstop dressage, and it's obvious to me that this was an act of cruelty— Prince has slightly mixed feelings about fences and can be a little sticky, and at one point I simply booted him over the last element in a low triple combination. My sheer size magnifies the dismal picture. As I watch myself turn off the line of fences and come down the long side of the arena toward the camera, I can see that my feet are level with the pumping trapezoids of Prince's knees and that my upper body looms over him like some monstrous bag of laundry with a helmeted head on top. I want to get under the sofa. Either everyone is too polite to say anything or they are all too busy grieving over their own performances, but for fifteen long minutes I think that it's time for me to quit riding and maybe learn to play mahjongg. Isn't that what women in their fifties are supposed to do?

We move on to the next video, which is of Ruth riding a difficult dressage test at some far-off competition, probably somewhere down south, since the land is flat and the light is, too—indiscriminate and free of shadows. Her big, muscled horse clearly knows his business, and Ruth carefully gives the impression that the horse is running the show and doing the movements pretty much on his own initiative—he *wants* to change his lead every two strides of canter, and he pirouettes around his back end with the air of a horse who has recently come up with rather a good idea. The only real clue as to who is operating the levers is that his ears tilt steadily back toward Ruth, who wears a flat-topped bowler, a black shad-belly jacket, and white gloves like a waiter's. This stately, dressed-up image is in complete opposition to the movies we have made of ourselves. It's demoralizing and frustrating—if she just rode a little less well, we might be able to figure out what she is doing. I do notice that Ruth is sweating mightily—the band of her high white collar is getting darker from the top edge down—and this is gratifying.

By unspoken consensus, the horse talk stops at the dinner table and we all seem to revert to our normal public selves. The big table is a nice place to sit, since it is next to a window that looks out toward the mountains; the spring light lingers so we can just make out their backbones as we start to eat. The conversation is general and friendly and curiously professional, as if we would all like a little distance from the day's events and the resulting videos, and we spend much of the meal talking with unusual enthusiasm about the state's environmental regulations. This is a topic even ordinary Vermonters are thoroughly knowledgeable about, and by the time we are done the mountains are gone and the windows have turned into inky mirrors.

The next day—and it may be just a coincidence—I am assigned to a larger horse. His name is Dr. Denton, and I recognize him right away as being Prince's turnout buddy from the day I rode him for the first time. Dr. Denton comes out of his stall a little boisterously, his head up and his feet restless, and he displays his Thoroughbred heritage by objecting to almost everything. Many horses with Thoroughbred blood in them do this as a matter of principle, as if they heard somewhere that the breed is fiery and intractable and feel an obligation to keep the rumor current. It's not particularly disturbing, but it surprises me when he does not get over it and start to settle down after a few minutes. If anything, he gets worse, as if I really were disturbing him. I try putting a firm hand on his shoulder to see what he will do. *What is up with you?* I silently inquire of Dr. Denton, who has his head up in the air and is swinging his haunches. He pauses to take note of my query, and my firmness, and becomes momentarily calmer, but continues to look at me anxiously out of the corner of his eye.

Jeanette, passing down the aisle, explains that Dr. Denton has been off work because he's been intermittently unsound, which means that he's been standing in his box more than usual, and been ridden less than usual, in the hope he will get better. This necessary rest has bottled him up and made him touchy and opinionated. Jeanette and I watch him for a long moment—Dr. Denton stomps and waves his nose—and then she suggests that I longe him first, before I get on, just to get the first layer of nonsense out of his system.

He's a big bay horse with a long neck and surprising reserves of physical grace, and at first he dances on the longe with a manic, graceful energy that is deeply pleasing to witness. He's good at being a little fierce, and he enjoys it, and I am actually mildly disappointed when he gets tired quickly and knocks it off—for those five minutes he is about as fully alive as a horse can be. But as he settles down and tends to business, he looks somehow wrong to me: His nose is wrinkled, and he seems balled up and not perfectly even. I can't locate this as an unsoundness, exactly, but more a problem with his general presentation. His top line—that curiously expressive run of horse from ears to tail—has a thick, stiff, slightly rumpled quality where it ought to be loose and free. He looks like he might like to buck but doesn't, which makes me remember the first time I met him, with his toga askew and his face bespattered with the residue of too much partying. It's hard not to wonder whether he is just naturally endowed with a larger-than-average dose of equine delinquency.

Once I'm on him, I'm surprised to find that Dr. Denton has certain psychic abilities—he proceeds around the arena relying on tiny cues and even tinier brain waves, and it's easy to override him. Some horses are like this. It's not always a function of sensitivity per se— all horses are about equally sensitive—so much as it's a defensive preference for understatement. Gem had this, and, even though Dr. Denton moves and thinks differently from her, he seems to be operating at about the same level of reactiveness as she did. Like Gem, Dr. Denton doesn't want me to *tell* him anything, but to offer up instead a small mental whisper, phrased as a suggestion. If I do try to *tell*, or insist on anything, he balks; he uses this balkiness as a tool to control me. I actually like this touchy, grouchy quality, since it lets me figure out exactly how unobtrusive he wants me to be. But it's also a communication technique that could invite roughness—more riding and not less—and I can tell that he's interested in luring me into making this mistake. Yet if I ride him on brain waves alone, buttressed occasionally by a few minor suggestions, I discover that he is not really delinquent at all but actually has many pluses; once we establish that less is more, he offers me an even, light feel in my hands and straight, comfortable strides. His canter to the left is particularly pleasing—not at all quick, and surprisingly easy to relax into. We are getting more than a few presentable transitions—walk to canter, canter to trot, trot to working trot, trot to halt—on psi alone.

I am happy with all these arrangements until we canter to the right. Weirdly, I don't sense any trouble coming. From his swinging walk, I propose a low, swinging canter on his inside leg, mostly by just thinking about the little back-legs jump of a canter departure and by flexing him a little to the inside so it will be easy for him to break that way. But as soon as I broach the subject, he begins pulling, and he really pulls in earnest, hurting himself with the bit and blaming me, and he slices to the inside, apparently avoiding some tiger who lies in wait for him along the rail. When I don't release him, he gathers the considerable strength in his neck and tries to drag the reins through my fingers; he then collapses forward, and his head disappears between his front legs. He isn't bucking, but it's a classic buck position. I realize almost too late that I'm in danger of sliding down this neck and landing on my chin, so I trade off, release the rein, and sit back so this doesn't happen. Dr. Denton is disappointed. This is a good trick, and it has obviously worked before, and as we reassemble our reins and seat and general composure I can feel him stiffening against me. He's mad now, and he has arrayed his personal army against the right canter departure, and his policy is that it's not going to happen.

It's hard not to wonder if he really is in pain somewhere, but he'd cantered perfectly well to the right on the longe line. We try again, and Kathie coaches me through it as best she can, but there's something tired in her voice, something resigned—she seems to know that nothing good will come of the exercise. "This is a new thing he's been doing lately," she says, implying that, prior to this, he was perhaps doing other things. After the fourth attempt she tells me to give up, and I canter him once, successfully, to the left, just to discourage in him the idea that he never has to canter again at all. He's tense, but reasonably obedient. As we come back to walk after a stiff but otherwise sensible circuit around the arena, I take a feel on the rein and ask him again—*What is up with you?*— and Dr. Denton responds to this inquiry with a dull and unresponsive blankness that actually unnerves me far more than his active resistance did. He does not like being queried; for the moment, he does not like me, even though he liked me fine just a few minutes ago. It's hard not to think that some small but important knob has gotten twirled on this horse, and this adjustment has turned him into the kind of animal, familiar to me, who is predisposed to eruptive, stubborn, transitory ideas. Later Kathie tells me in a semiconfessional way that Dr. Denton was bought for the school string but does not have the right physique or temperament for it. She adds, a little sadly, that one person, riding him the same way every day, could probably keep him sane and sound, but he lacks the resiliency of a Prince.

Within hours, my imagination is flooded with fantasies about Dr. Denton: I will buy him or lease him; I will learn his preferences; I will reschool him; I will solve his every problem; he will win important competitions. I know this is pure idiocy, but this is what riding is about: redemption, rectification, and repair, the three R's of the entire enterprise. After all, given enough time with Gem, I was able to slowly transform her and make her truly wonderful, and I yearn for this level of intimacy again. As we progress through videos and dinner, the movie running in my head takes precedence and becomes more elaborate and detailed: I imagine him wending his way toward me, whuffling in that way horses have of signaling they are not afraid; I see him accepting reassurances and discipline; I see him working calmly in a large, even circle, slowly bringing his muscles and his mind back into alignment and coherency. I imagine him learning to trust me and, like Gem, gradually revealing his essence for my acknowledgment and shy approval. We will cover all the old, absorbing, and important ground together; we will overcome; we will succeed and be famous. It's silly, but the pull of the scenario is muscular, and I have no power to resist it.

EIGHT

NOBODY SEEMS TO KNOW MUCH ABOUT THE PAIRING OF HORSE to rider, even though the act of pairing up may be the single most important thing in the riding world. In hunter and equitation competitions, judges are supposed to consider the suitability of horse to rider when they mark their cards, but this is mostly a size thing. But if size is what really matters, then Prince and I are obviously unsuitable even though we are on excellent terms; Gem, with her heft and stature, was clearly meant to carry a large rider, but there were many years when we did not suit each other well at all.

True pairing is an accumulation, and begins with a wordless and subterranean knowledge of what will likely happen around a particular horse. The rider slowly registers and then anticipates how an individual animal lifts her feet, steps over, announces pain, and peruses her agenda. On some level, whether intentional or not, the rider absorbs a horse's *style*. Are horses stylish? Yes—stylish and stylized—and there are real differences, from animal to animal, in their ways of being and how they deliver themselves to their handlers. Gem, for example, was a royal pain, but she was a royal pain in a very particular way: She wriggled and bounced, but she did not bite or kick. The longer I worked with her, the more detailed was my inventory of her tics and specific gestures—when I placed the saddle on her wide white back, she tucked her nose sharply toward her chest, once, and turned on her left front foot; she always pivoted to the right when I approached to mount; she always nodded when I brushed her mane. If she didn't do these things, she was sick.

That doesn't sound stylish, but more like Skinner-box behavior with all its rhetoric about stimulus and response. And it's very true that horses—unlike cats, say—are very amenable to straightforward behavior modification. You can use bribery and systematic cues to teach a horse to bow, back, shake hands, or do any other movement that can be broken down into small components. In her youth, Gem had been taught to ring a bell on cue and to paw the ground when asked how old she was. The result was that she rang imaginary bells and pawed whenever she sensed that something was expected of her that was even slightly outside the ordinary; worse, she did this with depressing reliability well into middle age, without reinforcement, and even in the face of my ongoing disapproval. These are tricks and have no value. But Gem's true style— her fretfulness, her energy, her physical courage—was an overriding theme that transcended bells and counting. Just the way we can recognize a friend from a distance by the way she turns her head or touches her chin, the same holds true for horses. Pairing is well under way when you can spot your horse, not by her markings, but by the posture she assumes in and toward the world.

For pairs to really stick, there must be reciprocity. My encounters with Gem in the pasture and on the longe line had shown me that she was more than merely difficult and squirmy—she was genuinely and abnormally sensitive, always looking for an opportunity to relieve her ongoing discomfort. Once I understood this, it became clear that, with Gem, the answer to almost every difficulty lay in subtraction, removal, and reversal. I never forgot that if I wanted to catch her I had to remove her halter, and that her best moments with her rider seemed to happen when I stayed off her back. My job was to take this metaphor and use it relentlessly, turning it into something concrete and real. This isn't easy with horses—they don't manage abstractions well.

But horses do manage nouns, and Gem looked upon her bridle, in particular, as a noun it was necessary to get upset about. Putting one on invariably involved a lot of head lifting, eye rolling, and attempts to score a few hard points off my feet. She wasn't all that delighted about saddles, either, and pivoted like a wind vane as soon as I lifted one, but the saddle business somehow seemed less urgent and more generic; once it was on, she forgot that it was there. The bridle was different: Even after I'd managed to get it in place, all her bridle-related behavior remained wildly erratic—she snatched, panicked, stopped, and exuded a diffuse and dangerous absence of composure. She would lean heavily on the bit and bore, but in the next moment would interpret my contact with her mouth as a signal to slam on the brakes or go backward. Or she would accept the contact for a little while, almost happily, and then begin running through my hands with her head in the air so I could not stop her. I had always ridden her in what I assumed was the very mildest of bits, a plain soft-rubber affair, but something about it, or something I was doing, made her change her ideas about it with each passing moment. I thought about the day I removed her halter and began to wonder: What if we dispensed with the whole business of bridles altogether?

Pulling this off wasn't easy, and in retrospect what I did was pretty stupid. I began by showing up in the pasture one day with all the usual harmless stuff—longe line, halter, longe whip—and also something new: a hard-plastic bucket. This last item puzzled her, but we looked at it together, and she verified that it wasn't red; Gem was prone to sporadic and pointless outbursts over a certain red bucket we had around the place. Even though my books assured me that she could not tell red from any other dark, saturated color, she obviously could—even at a considerable distance, she could easily distinguish the horrible red bucket from the acceptable dark green one, which, except for its color, was completely identical, right down to the date and place of manufacture. So I prudently brought the green one, and, after we established that it was empty, she indicated that it would be fun if I would fill it up with food for her. There was never anything wrong with Gem's appetite.

Keeping the bucket handy, we played the halter game and circled on the longe and practiced going into canter whenever I said *hup* and back to trot again whenever I said *ola*. A short, hard *ho* meant "stop." She wouldn't walk on the longe—I had never figured out how to convey the idea of it, and she had an impure, hurried, rather ugly walk that neither of us enjoyed—but these other gaits and the words that went with them were now perfectly stored in memory. The fun of it, I think, was the same fun that humans get from Mother-May-I or a game of freeze tag: How hard can we manipulate the rules before the whole thing falls apart? If nothing else, Gem was a stupendously alert horse, with a vestigial but improving sense of fun, but I doubt it ever crossed her mind that she was being obedient. It was simpler than that: She grasped the rules, she liked them, and she moved up and down the register of movements happily and promptly, wearing that same gratified expression that had surfaced the day we invented or perhaps discovered this game.

After a few rounds of play, I snapped a lead rope on either side of her halter, knotted them into rough-and-ready reins, and got the bucket. We confirmed, once again, that it was empty. She expressed, once again, a bit of disappointment that this was the case. I stood on it; she pivoted, snorted once, and began to back away. I got off, moved it, and got up on it again, and this time she went forward. Again I moved the bucket; she went backward. We did this for quite a while, sawing back and forth over about twelve feet of real estate, until it became obvious, even to Gem, that I really was going to stand on a bucket next to her left shoulder, and I was going to do it even if it took all day. She grumbled mightily but at last stood more or less still, and more or less in one place.

In a quick instant I was on, and Gem, thoroughly startled, was off and running. This was not at all a good development, but I instinctively said *ho* and reined her in. This time, however, there were no working reins connected to the usual hardware; only the ingrained habit of *ho* averted complete disaster. She slowed down, and at the same time my two lead ropes put pressure on the noseband of her halter. This noseband, to my surprise, actually got her attention—she leaned on it very briefly, testing it, and immediately discovered that it didn't hurt. She halted, puzzled, and waved her ears. She was thinking, and I exploited this unusual moment by turning her—Gem would always turn—back onto the familiar round longe track that we had worn into the grass. Here even more habit kicked in: She knew this place, and knew exactly what had always happened here, and to my surprise within a few minutes we could *hup* and *ho* and *ola* with the best of them, bareback and without a bridle.

The ropes offered up a strange sensation: It felt like I held her piebald face securely in my two hands, without variation or resistance, and she was suddenly present to me the way the normal horses I'd ridden were present with a bit that suited them. She didn't lean or hurry or pull the lead ropes through my fingers; instead she found the noseband, greeted it, and waited alertly to see what it had to say. I was new at riding with thick cotton ropes for reins, so the connection was a little blunt and rudimentary, but it was definitely there—she began to step forward into the halter with the kind of confidence that I knew was genuinely desirable. She was, as my various horse books liked to say, *in the bridle*, even though she wasn't wearing one. I decided to ignore this contradiction and settle for the plain fact that I *had* something, and that it was something I wanted, something elastic and alive and forward, something quintessentially Gem.

The downside of this risky enterprise was my own unsteadiness—her gaits were bouncy, I had no stirrups, and I wasn't doing much of a job of sitting still. As the minutes passed, my sloppiness began to worry her, and she got a little quick and rough, perhaps in the happy expectation that I might fall off—somehow, despite everything, I had yet to actually get dumped by her, and as a practical matter this was something I wanted to avoid. It was time to declare a victory and retreat, but as I slid down her shoulder and looked at her, I saw that she was suddenly being very peculiar, making mouthy, muttering, chewing motions as if she were looking around for a bit that wasn't there, or perhaps had a bee sting on her upper lip.

I didn't know it then, but this mumbling, accompanied by a glazed and curiously inward expression, was an actual signal. I couldn't classify it, because I'd never seen it before, but it's widely understood to be a gesture of submissiveness. Foals and low-ranking horses use it to deflect aggression from larger and more dangerous animals, but what it means between horse and rider is far more nuanced. The demands humans and horses make on each other are different, and these *don't-hurt-me* faces acknowledge that something about those demands is now understood. So yes, the expression is one of submission, but with a twist: It is the face horses make when they are in the mood to bargain, listen, make a deal. Some horses can even take offense if you do not pause to acknowledge that a face has been made. In retrospect, though, it was probably a good thing that I didn't pause and acknowledge or do anything else out of the ordinary, since I didn't know what I was looking at. If I had known, I might have turned smug or triumphant or been tempted to press my advantage; because I was ignorant, I didn't realize there was advantage to be taken. Instead I went the other way. Within a week—in a continuation of my discovery that removing equipment did more good than putting more equipment on—I switched Gem to a bitless bridle, a gentle and easygoing item called a hackamore.

Some of the people who were familiar with Gem's repertoire of quick, demented behavior made it quite clear they thought this was a step in the wrong direction, but it solved two problems right away: First, I could now bridle her without having an uproar, since she didn't notice when I put it on, and, second, as long as I behaved well, she never once questioned its authority. Over the next few months, I learned that the bone at the front of Gem's nose had real nuances and could be manipulated with the same careful subtlety as the inside of most horses' mouths. She reached for my hands, and settled into them comfortably, and even as I enjoyed this new smoothness and control, I burned with secret shame. For two years, I'd been inflicting pain, all of it unnecessary. I hadn't meant to, but I wasn't off the hook—intentions don't matter. It was obvious that even the fattest, softest, and kindest bit that money could buy could put her in a dismal and hopeless frenzy.

It was only after this discovery that the quality of her resistance to me began to change. She still behaved erratically sometimes, but she also accepted that I really was going to groom her, that I had a right to handle her feet, and that, if I wanted her to go down this trail rather than that one, I was qualified to make that decision. She stood still, at least some of the time, and no longer offered up pointless and explosive shifts in speed. At first, this actually worried me a little. I wondered whether she was tired, or perhaps needed veterinary attention—maybe this mouth thing she had started doing meant that she had used the rubber bit as some sort of pacifier or, as one of my books said, that something was the matter with her teeth. The vet came and filed off a couple of minor points and edges, but it didn't stop the transformation—she was still a handful, but was now a curiously compliant one. I continued to tiptoe around her with deference, and she still demanded deference from me, but something in the pitch of her hysteria had changed. She had periods of being interested, peaceful, and almost normal. After a year, I switched her, without fanfare, to a full-cheek snaffle bit that she let me slip in her mouth without resistance. She liked this bit and trusted me to handle it carefully, which was now possible to do because she wasn't acting like a lunatic. It was a moment of shared relief: The argument that had once consumed us both was finally settled. But the best part was that now, on some basic level, she was genuinely tamer, and when she was turned out in one of the pastures a long way from the barn I could bring her in by inverting one of the water buckets beside the gate, climbing aboard, and trotting her bareback up the dusty driveway.

NINE

ADULT WEEK RUMBLES ON, AND I SEEM TO BE BOUNCING around from horse to horse—a privately owned mare named Kitten, who is green and rough-gaited but who seems otherwise full of good intentions, and a school horse named Coach, a refined but very grouchy bay I have ridden once or twice before and have always secretly detested. I find I still detest him—he is stiff, hard in my hands, tiring, and confusing because he lacks Prince's responsiveness—but to my mild surprise I find that he is actually a better horse than I remembered. When I mention this to Kathie, she looks approving. "It's because *you're* getting better," she says. "He fights you less because you make more sense to him." It's possible she's right: I find that I can do almost presentable transitions between gaits on him, especially between walk and canter, and when he steps up into that first, round stride it seems to me, momentarily, that Coach is made of air.

But I've also spent most of Adult Week watching other people's horses—almost all the other riders have their own—and in the fullness of time I have become particularly fond of watching Railund, a massive Dutch warmblood. This term, *Dutch warmblood*, is both a breed and a designation—the stud books and registries for these horses are open, but only to animals who can pass a rigorous evaluation called a *keuring*. The idea behind these open registries is to allow people to carefully crossbreed horses—Thoroughbreds with Percherons, Irish hunters with Morgans, Arabs with Oldenburgs, and other selective, ingenious combinations—to get animals who are sane and sturdy and elegant, suitable for the top levels of competition. The funny name is actually logical, since warmbloods occupy the middle ground between the light, free-moving hot-blooded horses—Arabs and Thoroughbreds—and the steadier cold-blooded ones, mostly draft horses and the heavy carriage breeds. And of course, once you have a bunch of nice-looking warmbloods around the place you can start breeding them to each other, and soon enough a distinct and useful type emerges. As a group, they are heavy, strong, and beautiful, endowed with steady minds, hybrid vigor, and the expensive, correct conformation you see mostly at big shows and in horse magazines.

Railund has the warmblood aura in that he is beautifully proportioned in an ironclad, overbuilt way—large feet, thick bones, big chest, and powerful neck and haunches—but what I like best about him is his self-possession. Along with his rightness of shape, he also seems to have a rightness of character, since he is being ridden not by his owner, but by a novice named Judy who is as small for him as I am big for Prince—her heel falls just a few inches past the middle of his substantial barrel. Her legs are almost useless; to get him to trot, she taps him primly with a little stick. He registers this tap and serenely does what he has been asked to do, and his trot is naturally large and cadenced. Railund is careful with Judy, and he goes around the arena obediently if a little absently, his big Teutonic mind on other things. And despite what looks to me like very careful training and spectacular breeding, there is nothing at all fussy about him, nothing petlike, nothing easily insulted. Instead he exudes a kind of peaceful dignity, and steps up into canter with a steadiness that seems specifically engineered to accommodate Judy's relative lack of experience. Each time I see him do this, I become more impressed. Railund's owner is also among us, riding a different horse, and she has seen me watching him covetously. On Friday, the last day of the session, she generously offers me a chance to climb aboard.

There is something demoralizing about a horse who knows a lot, since there is only one place to put the blame. Railund, who was so settled and unthinking with Judy, reacts to me much the way Prince used to, crookedly and with his jaw set firmly in concrete. Obviously, this is something I invite and trouble I am myself causing, and this is not happy news. Railund proceeds around the arena with a determined and long-suffering blankness, rightly denying accountability, even though I am trying desperately to send him straight and forward, madly turning up the volume on all the things I have recently learned from Prince. It does a little bit of good but not much, since we are still dribbling around crookedly in his big trot making a mess of things. Worse, I can't really feel what's going on with his big hard body, since he does not have Prince's elasticity or responsiveness; all I can pick up on my radar is that I annoy him in a distant, slightly dismissive way. But I can't be sure even of this, since he mostly offers up a European density, an accented aloofness, that I don't quite know what to make of. Kathie teaches: "Don't let him say that to you, that was rude. Get on him with that outside rein and send him straight. He's leaning on your inside leg, so don't get sucked into leaning back—he'll do that. Bump him off with your heel, give him a pretty good tap, that's it. Say no. Now straight, straight, straight. You need more horse and less hand— more leg, and less of everything else. But don't give up—hold him on the outside. Live there. Don't let him escape, and don't soften until he knows you're really there, and then he'll be respectful.

Send him forward. Straight, straight, straight." I watch this session later on a video, and it amazes me what a difference in size will do. We are imprecise and out of sync and Railund looks extremely bored, but I somehow manage to look almost presentable—steadier, more relaxed, and deeper in the saddle. His natural carriage helps me set up a firm base of operations on his thick, muscled back, and the subject of cruelty does not come up. We are not a pair, but we are *suitable*. I know this is borrowed glory, but I'll take it.

One of the happy secrets of the horse world is that there is always some horse who needs to be ridden and some rider who needs a horse, and it is possible, with a little flexibility, sound administrative work, and careful matchmaking, to get these elements in alignment. It is even possible to have a long and interesting riding career based on this mechanism—you needn't actually become an owner. Technically, Gem was not mine; nor was my sister's horse, Tilly, hers. Of the six horses I have worked with seriously in two-thirds of a lifetime, there were only two I legally held the deed for. Sometimes these exchanges come about through convenience—an owner goes away to college but wants the animal kept sound and useful, or a horse needs to be kept fit if he is going to be sold. Other times they arise from sadness—a novice or timid owner is demoralized or frightened and needs assurance that a horse can, after all, be ridden. Or, as with Railund, a valuable and elegant horse is offered simply out of generosity—it was obvious to everyone at East Hill, including Railund's owner, that I could not go on riding Prince indefinitely. Railund was big and sturdy and mentally sound, the reasoning went, and I was not likely to do him any harm.

With borrowing privileges come certain responsibilities, and they all seem to involve a wheelbarrow. There are plenty of mysteries operating in the horse world, but the wheelbarrow is not one of them; everywhere you go, there is an infinite amount of mucking out to do, and mucking out, like housework, does not stay done. It has certain Sisyphean properties, and there is not much you can bring to the process to make it interesting. Even though each horse dirties a box stall in an individual way, each horse only has one way to dirty it, and once you've mastered that horse's pattern of where the mess will be—whether it is buried or out in the open, where the wet spot is, and how much poop will likely be deposited in the water bucket—there's nothing more to be done with that knowledge except to go get the wheelbarrow and rectify it. It's easy to see why cleaning stalls is a form of coinage—working students muck stalls in exchange for lessons, boarders muck stalls in exchange for a reduced monthly rate, and horseless riders muck stalls in exchange for access to someone they can ride.

Railund was well worth the labor. From the moment I got on and experienced his large, patient gaits, I knew he could do wonders for me. A made horse—a term that refers to an animal who has been taught to go well, even with an iffy rider—can quickly become a mentor by conveying how things ought to feel and ought to be done. Railund's composure was partly derived from his breeding and partly from his excellent upbringing; whatever the source, he trucked around the indoor arena with fortitude, Kathie teaching me to ride him forward, forward, forward in his massive, springy trot. Once we got *forward* at least partly established, the problems of getting him straight seemed to disappear with amazing ease: He rounded his back, settled evenly on the bit, and, for at least short periods of time, gave me the lifted, breathtaking feel of semicollection. This feel, when it arrived, was as if a door had been opened into a long, bright gallery with sunlit windows; I was now free to ride down this promenade with my attention firmly fixed on the rhythm of its details and the alternating pairs of legs that always manifested as bands of light and shade. It was a moment of intense synesthesia—the thump of each diagonal pair of legs was actively architectural, bringing with it a sense of tunneled enclosure but no claustrophobia. I could never sustain it, of course—whenever this cadenced architecture arrived and surrounded me, I invariably stopped riding and let Railund slowly collapse into something harder, lower, and more ordinary—but he had given me something that would have been otherwise unattainable. Now, when I heard the terms *using himself* and *balanced*, I had a set of images specific to Railund's trot that I could attach them to. And they always looked like a long, wide hallway, cloisterlike, with arched, evenly spaced windows.

Riding sometimes happens this way. Even though teaching is a wordy enterprise, the business of being on a horse is not. Henry Wynmalen faces this problem honestly by invoking poetry: "It is true that one must, in teaching riding, try to explain to students the nature and manner of the aids one uses, and to a certain extent this can be done," he says. "But only to a limited extent. . . . The same word, in poetry as in prose, can have many intonations and many meanings. Just so in riding, where the same aid can be given an almost infinity of meanings and intonations, whereby in the end a veritable language, and a reciprocal one, comes into being between horse and rider." Dialogue is a key concept here, but so is the reference to poetry; good riding, like good verse, is at once precise and hard to pin down, since both call to life all sorts of things that can't be located on the page or in the arena. Huge quantities of intuition are required, and this may explain why riding can also find its way to the surface through visual images or through music—the deep source, I think, of the *kur*, or musical program ride. It is important not to snort dismissively at the phrase *the art of riding*, because that is exactly what it is.

Yet there is always a certain amount of trouble in paradise, and the trouble with Railund was his aloofness. He was glorious but dismissive; he was a horse unusually busy with himself, imperturbable, and difficult to reach. Grooming him made me sad, since I felt I was grooming a warm, glossy statue—he was perfectly quiet and obedient, and nothing I did made the slightest impression on him. He was even more distant to ride. Mechanically sound, he purred along nicely, but his self-reliance troubled me. As the weather improved and I could ride him outdoors in the big jumping arena, he made the transition without comment, which frankly surprised me. Most horses, after a long winter of working indoors, relish the prospect of getting silly when taken out into the breeze and the sunshine—the sight of the horizon can be profoundly inspiring—but Railund was not subject to transports of outdoor glee. Our first time out, he took a few moments to look around, but he did it with the air of a bored teenager who has been instructed to admire the Grand Canyon. We then went back to our labors, and he trucked around the outdoor arena with the same steady resignation he had shown inside.

"I don't think I'll ever understand him," I said to Kathie at the end of a lesson. "He's inaccessible."

"He can be," she agreed, "but he's really teaching you something."

I had to acknowledge she was right, and I felt grateful for the many unearned successes he had handed me, but what I couldn't explain to Kathie was my own desolation. I felt alone on Railund, and unnecessary. It occurred to me that maybe I was incapable of making use of a well-schooled horse, and this depressed me. All the horses I had ever succeeded with were, in retrospect, pretty junky—oddly colored, plainly shaped, and often bred by accident—and maybe these cheapo horses were the only ones I would ever be qualified to handle. One warm spring day, as I cooled and groomed Railund before putting him away, I paused to watch a student trying to put a slightly tangled bridle on a certain shabby and alert buckskin pony. It wasn't going all that smoothly—Prince was being generically unhelpful, waggling around like a puppy in the cross ties—and I left Railund momentarily to go help her out. He greeted me and sniffed my leather leggings, noting the scent of Railund without jealousy; horses do not understand the concept of monogamy. For my part, I frankly enjoyed his hot breath on my knees. Calling him back to attention, I untangled the bridle, slipped it on, and checked the fit, and as the student went away with him for her lesson, I envied her.

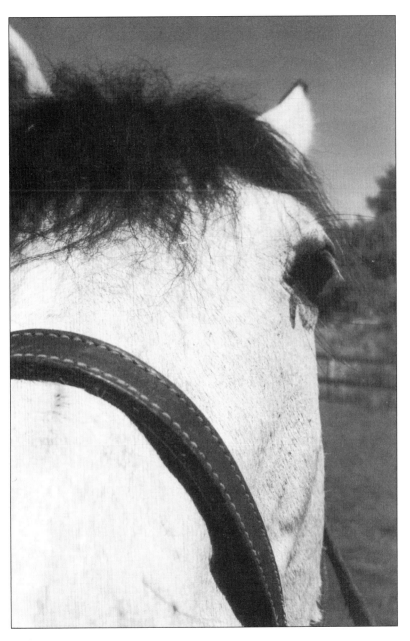

Prince. (Photo by Helen Husher)

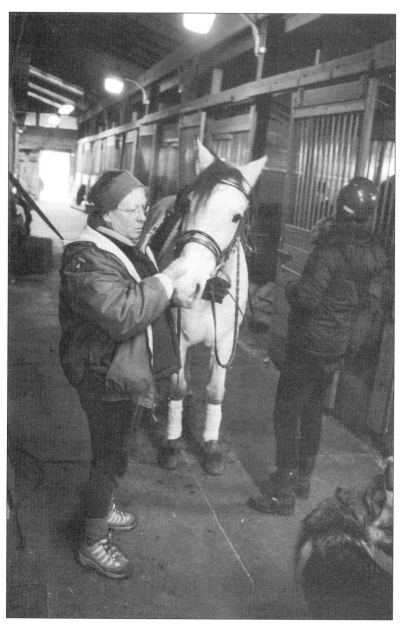

Kathie and Prince. (Photo by Helen Husher)

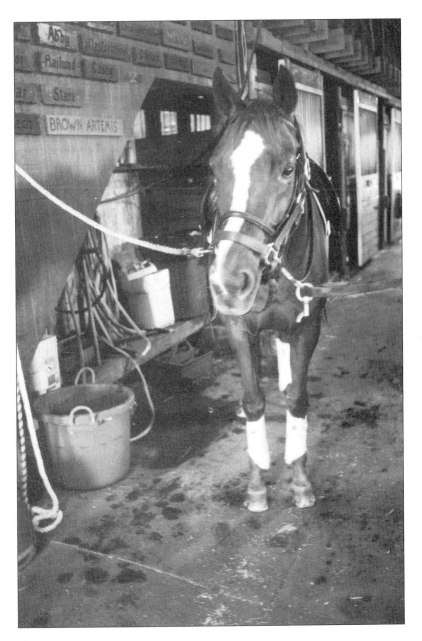

Reba. (Photo by Helen Husher)

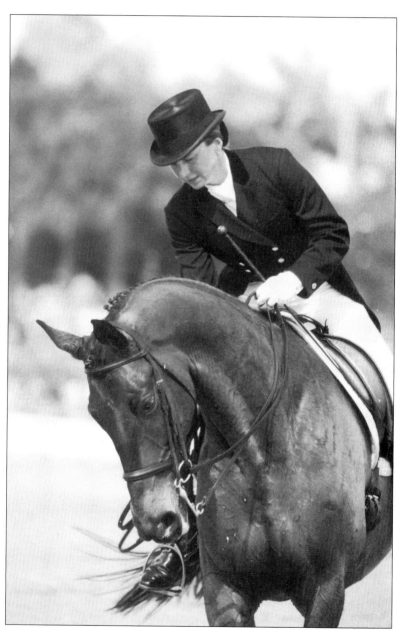

Ruth and Charmont. (Photo by phelpsphoto.com)

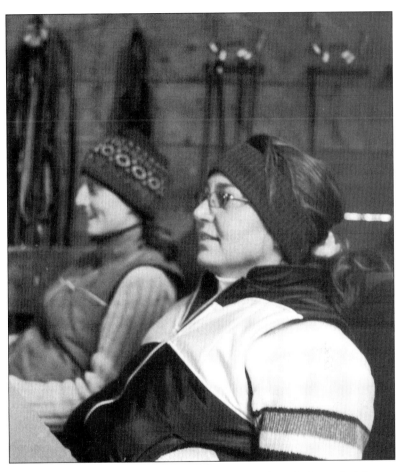

Ruth teaching a lesson. East Hill manager Meghan Maurice is on the left.
(Photo by Helen Husher)

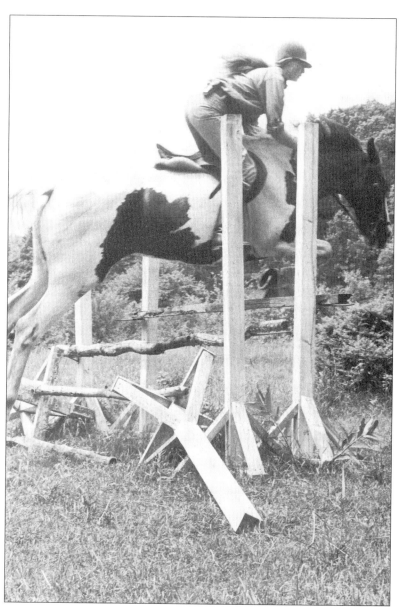

The author on Bones, about 1972. (Photo by Allan Pickman)

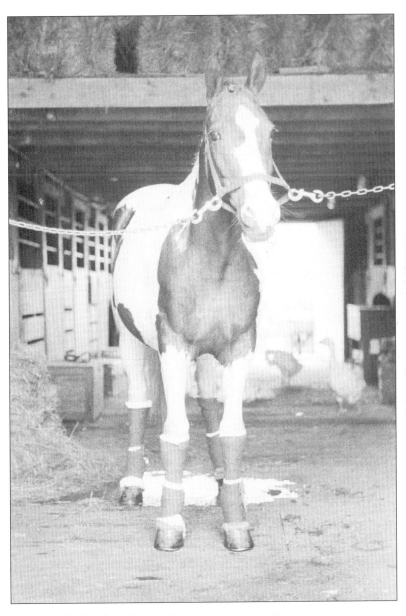

Bones braided and ready for a show. (Photo by Allan Pickman)

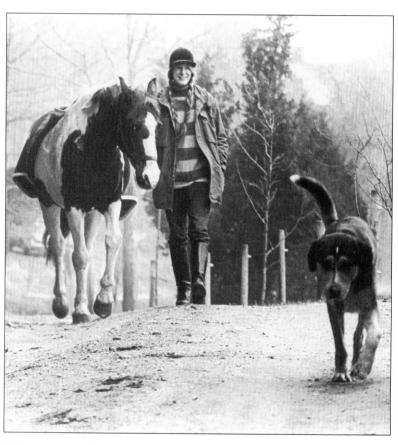

The author with Bones and Ranger, about 1975. (Photo by Allan Pickman)

TEN

"WHY," I ASK KATHIE, "ARE HORSES SO IMPORTANT? WHY IS IT that, if you like them, they become the only thing you really want to do?"

We are eating lunch together on a warm, early-summer day. The food is a good idea since it keeps Kathie, always a moving target, in one place. She looks thoughtfully at the innards of her BLT. "I think the people who do this, who come back to this day after day, are people who need a very high level of engagement," she tells me. "They have a lot of energy, they're smart, and they seem to get bored easily. They aren't the kind of people who would be content just sitting around doing nothing, because as you know there is always something to be done about a horse."

A horse, she goes on, is a complicated responsibility. It's not the feeding, the mucking out, and the mountains of labor so much as it is the way horses depend on humans to program their time and develop their abilities. "It's a mutual dependency thing. You put your horse in a program so he knows what's going to happen, what you expect from him, and this means you have to sustain that program and improve yourself all the time. You have to stay focused, you have to stick with it, and it's a lot of work." This exchange can wear down the uncommitted, but at East Hill it's the ticket you hand in at the door: "There are lots of barns that are more about fun, about having a good time with horses, playing with them, and maybe there's nothing all that wrong with that. And some horses seem to be okay with not being taken all that seriously, but a lot of them really aren't. They are not pets. It isn't healthy for them to get personified, to get treated as if they have human motives or human ideas, because they don't." Anthropomorphic expectations create confusion, and confusion leads to bad habits and equine spoilage. "We don't tolerate much of that. We ask our riders to respond to horses as horses, and to like them because of what they are."

Kathie admits that the barn sometimes loses students who aren't ready for, or aren't interested in, taking a serious line. But for the people who stay, this seriousness becomes the core of a community: "For most people, it isn't really about just having a horse, or they'd keep them at home. In many cases they could—there are several boarders who have nice barns sitting on their property. But they want to be part of a group, to be with people who have an interest in this long process of really learning to ride. I know I wouldn't enjoy it so much if I did it alone."

"But why do it at all?"

Kathie chews for a while before deciding it's safe to swallow. "For me, the drive to do it was always there, but I can't tell you where it came from. I grew up in Chicago, right in the city, where riding was really difficult, and all I wanted to do was go riding. I said, 'Take me riding, take me riding, take me riding.' I just about drove my poor parents crazy. And they did what they could—at first, I rode at a barn that was a converted parking garage, of all things, with these slippery cobblestone ramps between the levels, and the instructor was one of those people who shouted all the time, always yelling at everybody, and my father hated him. But they took me anyway, because I kept saying, 'Take me riding, take me riding, take me riding.' Then later, there was a much better place way out in the suburbs, and they would run lessons with twenty or thirty students in the ring, in this huge arena, and the instructors would be mounted and they would ride up beside you and teach you for a while, and then they'd circle away and teach somebody else. It was an interesting technique."

"It sounds sort of chaotic."

"You can't do it if you don't have good horses. They had very good horses."

"But that's not really an obvious thing, to grow up in Chicago and end up running a teaching barn in Vermont."

"No. But when the adults asked what I would do when I grew up, I'd explain that I was going to run a horse farm. I don't know how much I really believed it would happen, but eventually it did."

"You wanted it so badly. Why?"

"To me, all the time that I spend around the barn—well, no, let's put it this way. Every now and then you have a day when you get on a horse and the harmony just takes you, it's like listening to a choral group that's perfectly on pitch. It's just there, and it's so satisfying. There's nothing like it. Nothing. It makes you feel so good about what you're doing with your time, your life, your animals. That's maybe 5 percent of the time you spend on horseback. I can think of days when it happened. There it was—the flying change, or the half-pass, or the perfect canter, perfectly balanced. There was the half-halt where the horse understood that he was going to lift his shoulders. I remember, years ago, riding a horse who belonged to one of our boarders, and when I rode that horse, I never gave aids. I just thought about what we could do next and then we did it. It was like this conversation between us; it was like he was reading my mind. I would get an idea that we could canter, and there we were, cantering, and I realized I had to be careful what I thought. It was good. It was fascinating."

I instantly recognize this trancelike state and agree with her—getting wrapped in the magic of complete cooperation is like having a true dream or a long stretch of déjà vu. Horse ideas are not our ideas, but we can become privy to them if we mind our manners and keep the channel open, and sometimes horse ideas and our ideas silently merge so that everything we've learned—all that *correctness*—simply ends. These moments shine in a rider's memory as truthful and isolated and loaded with intuition. Riding stops being a sport, a discipline, or even a pastime and enters the realm of quiet revelation.

It was during one of these unmediated transactions that I first understood that Gem was not my pinto mare's real name. We were back in a normal bridle by then and things were going well, and one cold October day we were changing bends. This was not an exercise my horse really needed, since she was easily the most flexible animal on the planet, but we were doing it anyway. The books said to: "The lateral bend is correct when the horse is bent in the neck not more than in the whole body and when he flexes at the gullet," writes Alois Podhajsky, once the director of the Spanish Riding School, in *The Complete Training of Horse and Rider.* "A slight bend to the rein on which the horse is being ridden should always be demanded from a trained horse in an arena even when on a straight line." What the text could never fully explicate was that Gem loved and understood the bend, and knew much more about it than Podhajsky—each time I proposed a change in bend, she opened herself like a flower and became an even bigger horse, full of height and substance. After four or five switches, she requested, quite sensibly, that we change bends all day; I was finally asking her a question she knew the answer to. The exercise turned into a quiet trance of seeing what would happen next and where all this bending led to; for once, I wanted nothing from her beyond what she offered. Her name, I saw, began with *B*, because the happiness that radiated from her was about *B*—not *bend*, necessarily, but *B* for something in her talent, *B* for the placement of her feet on the dark, wet sand of the ring. *B* is for *big*, for *brave*, for *butter*—this sentence and this juxtaposition of bizarre ideas made perfect sense to me and left a deep impression. When she got tired we stopped, and it was a calm tired on a soft and intimate rein; my spotted horse looked around peacefully at a world that clearly began with *B*. From then on, I secretly called her Bones, because she had big ones, and after a while I couldn't hear her other name, Gem, without a little flash of irritation.

But other horses, horses I knew less well, had also done this for me. I returned to college in my thirties and became the student coach of a university riding team, and we all rode at a place in the suburbs of Boston, a superficially well-run barn that was for some reason infused with an unhappiness that I found sourceless and disconcerting. One night a week, I taught the lower-level team riders, and one night a week I rode myself with the more advanced ones, and I privately dreaded these expeditions because, even though the animals were well fed and fit, and even though the tack was clean, and even though the bedding in the box stalls was deep to the point of wasteful, the atmosphere around the aisles and in the arena was thick with misery. I could never pinpoint why—nobody yelled, nobody gossiped, nobody was to be found weeping behind the shed row—but something was wrong. Going there was like entering the family home of secret drinkers or perhaps a place where pit bulls chewed each other raw in a soundproof basement. The other team riders also noticed this dark uneasiness, but I couldn't bring myself to initiate a switch. Abbott was there, and there was no way I could do without Abbott, since Abbott was the antidote to all my reservations about the place and to my many reservations about life in general. Like Kathie's boarder horse, Abbott needed no aids, but simply responded without interface; he was never, technically speaking, obedient, since the question of obedience hardly ever came up. Abbott was there, and I was there with him, and together we jumped things because Abbott had a high opinion of jumping. He knew a lot about it and loved solving the spatial problems it presented, and he never chose to jump the same run of fences in exactly the same way. Sometimes he experimented and made what looked like a mistake, but it really wasn't, since he was exploring what could be done between the oxer and the combination, the combination and the angled gate. My job was to help him think and stay out of his way. It was also my job to know when Abbott was done with a particular set of obstacles and wanted something new—he resented jumping anything easy or anything he already understood, and he often took rails down if you insisted. After a while I knew better than to ask.

I snap back to the present and realize that I have been sitting in a stupor, my left hand holding a pickle in midair. Kathie completely ignores my long absence from the conversation and picks with contentment at the remains of her sandwich, which by now consists of lettuce litter and a few frayed potato chips. This moment reminds me that horse people, as a general rule, are amazingly talkative, but they also understand long silences. They tend to treat them as punctuation, and not a social emergency.

"They're all so different," I say.

"They are."

"And nobody agrees on who the good ones are."

"No."

"You would think after all this time we would know, that it would be the ones with a certain talent or the ones who look a certain way. But that isn't how it works." I am thinking of Railund, an excellent horse I don't seem to have any radar for, and Prince, who is unglamorous but agreeably transparent to me.

"There are some horses I just don't like, horses I don't like to be around," Kathie says. "That doesn't mean they aren't good horses, because a lot of them are, but they are good for somebody else." She pauses. "It goes by type, I think—Jeanette, for instance, can't ride a Thoroughbred. She makes them nervous, and they make her nervous. But of course what marks out a really skilled trainer or rider is the ability to get beyond these personal preferences and learn to read and develop every animal. The better you are, the less it matters." She is right, and I know she is right, but it's no fun being reminded.

A few days later, I ask Jeanette a lot of the same questions. The overall shape of her story is very different—Jeanette did not begin riding as a child and never had the fever-itch to be around the barn. Instead she began in her thirties because of her daughter Ruth, who at six was swung up innocently on one of Kathie's horses to see if she liked sitting there. She did, very much, and a long and complicated riding career began. Right from the beginning, it was a career that pulled Jeanette along in its powerful wake. At seven, after a year of lessons, Ruth was given the opportunity to bring a pony home to Jeanette and Con's farm in Berlin, Vermont, for the winter, in part to see if she was really willing to do the work, day in and day out, and to do it during a time of year when there wasn't much payoff in terms of saddle time. A young girl hauling water, which is heavy and slops all over and is quite cold in January, is almost overdetermined in its importance. Either the water is carried joyfully or it isn't.

Water was carried and Ruth was committed, and Jeanette said, "I realized I *had* to learn, because I had to know something about this. We could see where Ruth was going, but you don't let a young child start up with something like this without getting some education yourself." Then Kathie bought the initial tract of land in Plainfield that would eventually become East Hill Farm, although East Hill Farm, at first, was not on anybody's mind. "One summer Kathie asked us to come help her hay. We did, and we found out that another piece of land was available up here. So we bought it, but mostly as an investment—we had no idea, at the start, that we would all end up running a business together."

It was Con, Jeanette's husband, who came up with the idea to do a market study to see whether a teaching barn with an indoor arena—something Kathie had always wanted and something Ruth would need—was a viable proposition in central Vermont. "The survey work seemed to be saying yes, it could be a viable business," Jeanette says, "and so we went around the state checking out all the indoor riding facilities we could find to get ideas of what would work. And I think we looked at seven. Whether that was every indoor school in the state in the mid-1970s or not I don't know, but it was pretty close. Now there are twelve indoor schools in Washington County, and there are four just here in Plainfield." Plainfield is home to 1,286 people and, obviously, a growing number of horses.

But East Hill, Jeanette calmly concedes, does not really make any money. "The barn supports our own horses, but nobody draws a salary." Off-farm income keeps food on the table—Kathie's husband, Bill, is a forest manager, and Jeanette's husband, Con, is a consultant, a past state commissioner of human services and corrections, and not long ago made a credible run at being Vermont's governor. Ruth also makes a good living in her own right as a trainer and instructor. "But that's different," Jeanette says. "She offers a different kind of expertise, and to a different clientele, and she charges a lot more. We wanted to keep it affordable—the full legal name of the barn, you know, is the East Hill Family Riding Center. Choosing that name was a way of saying what we wanted to do, something we think is important."

This important thing, Jeanette explains, is the effect riding has on people's lives: "Dealing with horses is a true-to-life experience. It helps kids learn how to deal with responsibility, how to deal with disappointment, how to deal with success, and how to make a commitment to a long-term process." Watching students progress through the program is a satisfaction in its own right for Jeanette, since she knows that it's not possible to learn to ride without examining your faults and testing your resolve. "And it's more than that," she says. "You have to ask yourself—and we have asked ourselves—*What is it that kids really need?*" Here Jeanette goes off on what seems at first like a tangent, describing a conference she once attended with Con where this was the burning question; after a certain amount of groping and waffling around, the attendees found what felt like a working answer. "What they decided, in the end, was that kids need a relationship in their life that they can count on. That's very simple, and it's also true. I think it's something we provide here—strong human relationships."

It's strange to me that Jeanette has so many thoughts about the human relationships in the barn and so few about the equine ones, which to me have always been the essential and healing ones. But I also know she's right, since one of the qualities of East Hill is its welcoming and unsnobby ambience, its easy inclusiveness. It was the first thing I noticed when I came to the barn, and I still notice it with fresh surprise when a person I am not sure I know asks for a hand with bringing in a brace of horses or operating a pair of clippers.

Everyone, regardless of income or skill level, has a rough equality and an absolute right to exist. At East Hill this can be counted on, and its value is only enhanced because it's not often the case; barn culture, like corporate culture, varies greatly, from loose and sunny to competitive, stressful, over-regulated, and tragic. Unlike Jeanette, though, I only seem to register how it affects the horses, and I only see the value to the people when it's pointed out to me.

"Is it true," I ask her, "that you don't like Thoroughbreds?"

"It is," Jeanette says. "I don't get along with Thoroughbreds, because I want to be in control and so do they. It's probably because I learned as an adult—I worry about them running away or doing something unexpected. So I tend to use a heavy rein, and I have a hard time giving, and when you do that to Thoroughbreds they get pissed. And it turns into a circle—I don't want to give to them, so they don't want to give back to me. The warmbloods are so much more forgiving—if I hang on a warmblood, he's not necessarily going to do what I want, but he's also not going to go dancing and prancing all over the place, either. It's the temperament—warmbloods are selectively bred for temperament, and that's the temperament I really want. Even if I say I was never afraid, learning to ride as an adult, I do think learning to ride late was a factor. I don't want to worry, *Where's he going to go? What's he going to do next?*—and I really think it's because I didn't gallop bareback through the woods when I was twelve. Not having that to draw on makes me much more careful."

ELEVEN

SUMMER IS PROGRESSING AND I HAVE TURNED INTO A VOLLEYBALL, bouncing with a tight, airy *tang* among many horses, none of them Prince. It really is a weightless sensation—I have no one to moon over between my lessons and no real way to gauge my progress, although it does seem I am making some. Now, when I settle into the saddle, I sit deeper and move less; when I am confronted with a minor problem—a careless bit of bulge, a little stiffness—I can fix it on my own. There are one or two things about my behavior that Kathie no longer talks about, which means they have finally sunk into the silent pool of muscle memory, but at the same time I have entered a period of begging, almost childishly, to ride without stirrups. I recognize this right away as being part of an old reflex that insisted, *If things are not going well, take something away.* Stirrups suddenly seem to me to be a bad idea, restrictive and unnecessary and irritating. They seem designed only to push me up, away from the place I yearn to be, which is some elusive location inside the horse's rib cage, perhaps in the vicinity of the heart. It's my way of chasing the thing I am close to but can't quite get—the real dressage rider's deep, expressive seat—but I also want a certain informality to flavor the proceedings. I'm in an atavistic mood—perhaps I want, as Jeanette says, to be twelve again, and crashing bareback through the forest at an intemperate speed.

Enter Reba. She is a new presence in the barn, a chipmunk-colored Thoroughbred mare with a dished face, strange patches of bare skin around her large eyes, and a reserved, edgy alertness that demands deference without her having to condescend to threats or posturing. She feels alpha—a term for a high-status mare in a free-living group—yet at the same time defensively submissive around the humans, dropping her head as I groom her and making *don't-hurt-me* gestures with her delicate lips. She stands perfectly still under the brush but is not aloof; instead, she seems wary and excessively alert, protecting herself and taking stock. This unusual combination evokes quiet, respectful handling from her human keepers, as if she were made out of china.

Perhaps she is. When I ride her for the first time, I see she shares Prince's willingness to listen, but the quality of her attention is utterly different. Prince is always happy to do something new, but doing what you want is low on his list; Reba's responsiveness has a moral dimension, a desire to do things right, whereas Prince is playing his life for the laughs. Her obsessive obedience is almost embarrassing, since any questionable result, even if it's due to her various limitations, is never grounded in her resistance. She has no resistance. Reba wants order, certainty, and knowledge. I see immediately that she would be a very easy horse to ruin. I am careful with her, and everyone else is careful, too. "She's awesome," Kathie says, simply. This strikes me as an accurate and nontrivial use of an otherwise shopworn word.

Reba, I'm told, has been raced—she won quite a lot of money in her day—and retrained as a polo pony, and then tried for a while as a hunter, but despite these athletic experiences she is lopsided and surprisingly awkward, as if each new discipline were only half explained and ended up a source of worry and confusion. She can be challenging to ride—a disconcerting mix of speed and clumsiness—but her work ethic is the thing that saves her. On no other account is she a particularly attractive horse, since there is something underfed and ordinary about her general outline. Yet I sense she is not ordinary. New to the demands of basic dressage, she seems to grasp quickly that it is something specific, and is therefore worth paying attention to. Each time I ride her, I am painfully aware of the considerable weight of her seriousness.

Many things about Reba surprise me, but what's most noticeable is that, for such an edgy horse, she is strangely soothing to be around. When I go to catch her at turnout, she comes deliberately, fluttering her nostrils; when I lead her, she is so focused on my intentions that she seems to float magically at my side, as if I were not leading her at all but accompanying her on some important errand. Yet there is nothing smarmy about her, nothing craven; instead she allows her handler inside the bubble of righteous inquiry that she carries with her. It's a strange sensation, and perhaps a lot to live up to, but if Reba can do it, I figure so can I.

One final upside to Reba is her ignorance—she does not know more than I do, and it feels good to be on equal footing. She is not yet a dressage horse, and I find I can pay more attention to her because of this. I also fully appreciate that she knows *different* things: There are moments when I feel the characteristic *let's-go* Thoroughbred response that can pop out unexpectedly in horses off the track, the brightness and speed that Jeanette finds unnerving. I like it, and for some reason I associate these bursts of energy with her confused résumé—it is as if she sometimes needs to recapture her successful race-horse self before reappearing warily in the present. Or maybe that's too complicated, but there is nothing at all alarming about it. Instead she interests me, and one summer day I find myself just standing, watching, and thinking about Reba.

She doesn't fidget, and she doesn't look for something else to do. She waits, and she looks back.

Anna Sewall's *Black Beauty: Autobiography of a Horse* is sappy and dated and packed with only partially cooked ideas about horses, but it has an ethical dimension that reminds me of Reba. Reba, like that book's narrator, has grasped that there is something to be gained through the discomforts and demands placed on her by humans. Black Beauty tells us:

> Every one may not know what breaking in is, therefore I will describe it. It means to teach a horse to wear a saddle and bridle, and to carry on his back a man, woman, or child; to go just the way they wish, and to go quietly. Besides this he has to learn to wear a collar, a crupper, and a breeching, and to stand still while they are put on; then to have a cart or a chaise fixed behind, so that he cannot walk or trot without dragging it after him; and he must go fast or slow, just as his driver wishes. He must never start at what he sees, nor speak to other horses, nor bite, nor kick, nor have any will of his own; but always do his master's will, even though he may be very tired or hungry; but the worst of all is, when his harness is once on, he may neither jump for joy nor lie down for weariness. So you see this breaking in is a great thing.

Granted, this *great thing* does not sound like a whole lot of fun, but part of *Black Beauty*'s value lies in the recitation of human behavior from Beauty's perspective, which leads naturally and seamlessly into Beauty's judgment of his handlers. Yet despite its heavy irony, the above passage is actually a prelude to a description of some very good treatment—no sacking out or other horrors here—

and one of the reasons *Black Beauty* continues to shine in our literature is the decisive and sacrificial content of that final sentence. The entire narrative is built around the hero's absolute acceptance of the human agenda, and as the story progresses it is his excellent comportment that consistently saves him. So breaking in *is* a great thing; Sewall captures, with only a little bit of melodrama, the idea of willingness.

Almost all the horses in *Black Beauty* are willing, some of them to the brink of idiocy, in that they only resist when asked for more than they can give. Thus carriage horses, tormented by careless drivers, pull heavy loads of people and baggage until they collapse in the traces; small ponies jump steadfastly until the fence is simply too high. The refusal to go farther or jump higher is invariably answered with a drubbing, which raises the question of why this book is understood to be suitable for children. Captain, whom Black Beauty meets while working as a London cab horse, offers up the story of his experience as a cavalry mount. It's not a very nice story, but Captain tells it with enthusiasm—the charge, the hiss of bullets, and the execution of injured horses on the field of battle. Even Ginger, an edgy and defensive chestnut mare who is an emblem in the story for all suspicious and damaged horses, eventually learns to find gratification in her work—it becomes for her, however briefly, *a great thing.*

This depiction of willingness and its consequences probably explains at least some of the book's magnetic pull. We like to place our ideas about the assumed nobility of the horse inside a human frame, and I think we particularly like it when horses speak to us in the first person, explicating the equine point of view. Yet *Black Beauty* is also meant to make us uncomfortable. The author, a Quaker crusader for the welfare of horses, was on a mission to abolish the use of check reins—a piece of equipment that holds a horse's head unnaturally high—and to lecture the reader about kindness, temperance, and family values along the way. These parts of the book get old in a hurry—there are several long passages on the evils of drink and the importance of not working on Sunday—but the larger story still has tremendous momentum as the narrator moves from one owner to another, and it's done so well that we don't even object all that much when we run across a chapter called "Ruined and Going Downhill." We accept this overcooked diction because we understand that this is an epic, complete with the requisite demons, setbacks, and temptations; the story even ends with a recognition scene and homecoming straight out of Homer's *Odyssey*. Little Joe Green, an apprentice groom from Beauty's early days, does the required inventory of salient characteristics: "'White star in the forehead, one white foot on the off side, this little knot just in that place'; then looking at the middle of my back—'and, as I am alive, there is that little patch of white hair that John used to call "Beauty's three-penny bit." It must be Black Beauty! Why, Beauty! Beauty! do you know me?'" Beauty is home at last.

Talking horses run the gamut from Mr. Ed, whose trivial discourse is more like a nagging spouse's than anything else, to the title character in Leo Tolstoy's "Strider: The Story of a Horse," whose monologues are introspective, depressive, and unsettling. Strider, now old and lame, meditates on the shape his life has taken and its link to the human use of the possessive. The claims made by certain pronouns indicate to Strider that people are guided "not by deeds but by words. They like not so much to do or abstain from doing anything, as to be able to apply conventional words to different objects. Such words, considered very important among them, are 'my' and 'mine,' which they apply to various things, creatures, or objects; even to land, people, or horses. They have agreed that of any given thing only one person may use the word 'mine' and he who in this game of theirs may use that conventional word about the greatest number of things is considered the happiest."

Strider is puzzled by the perversity of this, but Strider himself is just as perverse in his own way. Addressing the herd, he describes his happiest years as those spent with a flashy and dissolute officer of the hussars. "Though he was the cause of my ruin, and though he never loved anything or anyone, I loved and still love him for that very reason. . . . You understand that lofty equine feeling of ours. His coldness and my dependence on him gave special strength to my love for him. 'Kill me, drive me 'til my wind is broken!' I used to think in our good days, 'and I shall be all the happier.'"

Lofty equine feelings are an artifact of the human imagination, but willingness is real. Why else would horses consent to being ridden at all? After all, it is in many ways against their interests and even their instincts, since the very place we humans want to sit—on their backs—is one of the places horses worry about the most. It is horribly vulnerable, being both a landing pad for tigers and a blind spot in their visual field. Horses can see backward and sideways, all along their flanks, and, except for a triangle of nothingness directly in front of them, they can see forward, but their riders are invisible—the only part of us they can see while we are mounted is our feet. This isn't really enough of our anatomy to take an intention reading, and what's more we often behave ominously up there, making mysterious, sometimes conflicting demands. Once we get off, we interfere with their social lives, strap them up with complicated equipment, tell them they must wait before they can scratch where it itches, and even shave off their whiskers—this last is a particularly unpleasant imposition, since horse whiskers, like cat whiskers, are an important source of sensory information. Yet horses are large and powerful and can run very fast, so they can easily pursue other options besides cooperation. Some of them do; most don't. This seems obvious and even trivial, but is actually wonderful—we do not think about the choices horses make because we are habituated to them.

As for Reba, she is now being ridden by a number of students, and her initial hypervigilance gradually blurs and softens. This says a lot about how she is being ridden, since in many lesson barns things could easily have gone the other way, but it's obvious as the weeks go by that the mare has come under the protective and probing sponsorship of Kathie's attention. Kathie tells me that Reba has an important role to fill in the teaching program, and I don't doubt this is true, but the way she talks about Reba is something of a giveaway—we discuss in depth her preferences and her knowledge and her mannerisms, and one day we even have a long and complicated conversation about how Reba acts when you enter her stall. The lessons, which on other horses were mostly about me, become mostly about Reba, and the vocabulary changes: "What we want," Kathie says, "is a signal, so she knows when what she's doing is what we want, that she's trying in the right direction, and you need to use your voice, say *good girl*, then give. That's right. Sit absolutely still. Support her with that outside hand, but just support her—what you want is to wait for her over there, wait for her to *fill up* that rein, just wait patiently for her to come down and get softer—more flexion, more flexion—and yes, that's right. Now give, open your fingers just a little, make sure you unlock your elbow. There. Say she's a good girl, and now wait again. It's going to feel rubbery, like a rubber band in the outside hand, and you wait for her to stretch it through, stretch it through the flexion. More flexion, more flexion, that's right; there's your answer; now say *good girl* and relax your hand. Keep talking to her, keep it going, keep her interested, ask for a little more. Good girl. That's right. Good girl."

Everything in the tone of this is new, and Reba, once quick and stiff and a little anxious, now takes only twenty minutes of careful riding to lower her head, slow down and open up her hurried trot, and gradually unlock her jaw. Her outline may still be a little flat along the top, and she may be a little too long, but her tempo is lighter and more definite, an improvement over her previous worried shuffle. Still, the new importance of this flexion business ruffles her up a little, and sometimes she bores down anxiously on the bit. When this goes on too long, we pause so that Kathie can cross the bright sand of the outdoor arena and play the thick jointed snaffle bit gently across the bars of her mouth, first on one side and then the other. Kathie then turns her head and stretches her neck, finding and resolving little pockets of stiffness. Reba droops her eyelids, absorbed by these new and obviously inebriating physical sensations. She leans into Kathie and seems to take inordinate pleasure in her presence, and sometimes interrupts the exercise to slobber on her sunburned arm.

TWELVE

WITHOUT BECOMING A QUAKER CRUSADER MYSELF, I UNDERSTAND that the work Kathie does with Reba is a great thing. It reminds me of something Ruth said in a different setting about a different animal: "He likes my program," she said, "and I like his." At the time she said this, I was thinking wrongly about what the word *program* really meant—I associated it with things like *regimen*, *system*, *approach*, and yes, even *correctness*. It does mean those things, at least on the surface, but when Ruth and the other skilled riders at East Hill talk about putting their horse in a program, they seem to be describing something far more potent than the progression of movements that a dressage horse must learn. It is not enough to put in the tricks—the pirouettes and lead changes and half-passes—because the tricks, on their own, are potentially meaningless and can even be destructive. What you are putting in, I see as the weeks go by, is more willingness, and it's a willingness nuanced by the wish, expressed by both parties, to do something difficult and interesting together. Xenophon, the Greek essayist and historian, was right: "What the horse does under compulsion," he wrote in *The Art of Horsemanship*, "is done without understanding;

and there is no beauty in it either, any more than if one should whip and spur a dancer."

Then, one windy and surprisingly chilly summer afternoon, Ruth sets aside some time to talk to me about her life with horses. Ruth is thirty-seven but looks much younger, with the neat, confident body language of a teenager. On this day, she also looks disheveled and relaxed—her summers on the home farm, she says, are what she needs to regroup after the rigorous competition schedule she maintains in Florida during the winter. "Here, the pressure's off," she says. "I can teach and school my horses and do all the same things I do down there, but it's not a fish bowl. In Wellington, I'm surrounded by some of the best riders in the country, and I want that, but it's intense and stressful. I need this." She gestures out the barn door toward the bright hills. "Here, if I want to, I can go for a trail ride."

Ruth says that, as a very young rider, she went about the business of learning with a terrible intensity that is not often seen in first-graders. "My mom never thought I'd be able to stick with it because I was such a nervous kid," she says. "And I was. Going to my lessons, I'd get sick in the car, and it wasn't at all about being afraid. I was never afraid. I got sick because I wanted to do it right so badly—I always wanted to do it better." This perfectionism was actually a little problematic; Ruth's first horse show was also Ruth's first encounter with an element in her character that drove her forward and held her back at the same time. It began when her teacher, Mary Ann McFaun, encouraged Ruth to go to a local show and enter in the lead-line class.

Now, the lead-line class is in some ways no class at all—young children on peaceful ponies are led serenely around at a flat walk. The performance dimension for the riders consists mostly of keeping both feet in the stirrups and not bursting into tears; if you can do that, you have a real shot at a ribbon. Since Ruth had been cantering and even jumping in her regular lessons, it should have been a laugher. For Ruth, though, the whole situation looked quite different. "We got to the horse show, and of course I'd never seen anything like it before," Ruth says. "I saw all the older kids riding so well and doing all these things I'd never done, things I couldn't do, and I just knew it, I knew I wasn't good enough. I wasn't ready to go into that ring, and I simply refused. I would not go." Coaxing didn't help, and so Ruth stood anxiously on the sidelines as a different child rode the pony she'd been slated to go in on, a child who had never even tried to ride before. He won the class.

"I decided," she says, "that I probably wouldn't let that happen again."

That first show was followed by many others where she did go in, but Ruth says her early career was marked by a nervousness that transcended ordinary precompetition jitters. "Even though I showed a lot and I did a lot of different kinds of competing—hunter classes and eventing and dressage and equitation up to Medal-Maclay—I just never really felt *prepared*." Some of this, Ruth concedes, was because she was not riding particularly nice horses. "I got to be a good rider because I was riding everybody else's junk," she says. "They were the leftovers—all the horses who wouldn't go over the jumps, the ones with physical and mental problems. I always had the tough horses, the cheap horses, the horses off the track, whatever we could find that I could make go around. It taught me a tremendous amount, but it also meant I was never completely sure what was going to happen."

This readiness, or the quest for it, may be one of Ruth's defining features, in keeping with her physical quickness and her squarish, stubborn chin. Oddly, she talks very little about winning—winning and being prepared are related, it seems, but they are not the same thing. "If you're going to go down the centerline," Ruth says, referring to the beginning of every dressage test ever written, "then you have to *know* certain things. Maybe you have to know that your horse is going to try to get behind the bit when you halt at X, and if that's the case then you really have to *know* that. Of course you also have to try to ride through that problem and make it better, but you don't pretend that it will not happen, because it probably will. And before you go down the centerline, you have to do everything you can to make it a good experience for you, the horse, the judge, everybody."

As it happens, one of Ruth's trips down the centerline was caught on a videotape that became part of a televised *Nature* special called "Horse and Rider." It's an interesting piece of footage, not because the ride is perfect—there are several rough moments that even an inattentive onlooker can see—but because the ride is about creating a good experience for a horse whose belief in goodness is in short supply. This horse, Charmont, is more proof that it is not enough to put in the tricks, since previous trainers had put them in with a vengeance, to his eventual ruination. One result of this rough treatment was that Charmont, despite his very advanced training, had earned a reputation for conduct so disorderly that, when he was delivered to Ruth's Florida barn, he came in a horse ambulance—it offered really good padding and meant that emergency equipment was right at hand. Ruth knew the horse was problematic before deciding to take him on, but the appearance of this piece of equipment in her stable yard really rattled her: "Here's this horse, all shackled up in there, and I thought, *oh my God, I've really done it now.* But at the same time, I didn't want to know anything—I didn't want anyone to tell me about his routine, or what he did, or what he didn't do, I just did not want to be told anything. I wanted to find out for myself." What she found, it seemed, was a horse who had been so wrongly and forcefully taught that he had become trapped, without choices or autonomy.

Early in the *Nature* segment, we see the problem: Charmont knows what is expected of him, and he fears it. Fear stiffens his joints and flattens his expression and makes him dangerously unhappy. Ruth's job, perversely, is to evoke his unhappiness and to greet its appearance with composure—at one point, Charmont rears and skitters with amazing power across the arena. Ruth skitters right along with him, a motionless and unpunishing essay in being *prepared* without being at all on the defensive. Her ground coach, the U.S. Equestrian Team veteran Jane Savoie, addresses the camera: "What makes Ruth such a gifted trainer," she says, "is that her priority is to relate to how the horse is thinking, and to not impose her thoughts on the horse." This looks and feels true—Ruth's entire posture is one of neutral acceptance—but when the disobedient episode is over, Ruth does impose at least one thought on Charmont. She visibly relaxes, gives him a pat, and puts him back to work again.

What the camera doesn't capture—what the camera was not there to see—is that by midsummer of that same year Ruth was going down the centerline on a transformed Charmont and competing in top company at Intermediate I, a level of competition that is not intermediate at all, but a slender notch below the level required for Olympic competition. "What Charmont taught me was to let go of mistakes, which was good for me as a competitor," Ruth says. "It's very easy to fall apart in a test—if you keep thinking about a mistake, then before you know it the test is over. I had to stay focused and ride for every point." This improved her work with her more consistent horse, Mastermind, who really did win. But competing isn't always about winning: "People kept asking me why I bothered with Charmont, why I moved him up to the Grand Prix, knowing I was going to always end up in the middle of the pack—they thought I was wasting my time. But Charmont kept me sharp and honest, and it was at least partly because of him that I understood what it meant to be *prepared.*

"The whole story about Charmont is a story about trust," Ruth continues. "He'll never be easy, and he'll never be over all his stuff, but people can ride him now, and he doesn't have panic attacks and rear and walk around. I did make a choice, though, and decided not to press him past the point where he could still be accepting. I could feel it; I could feel him thinking *Now we're coming up on the one-tempes*"—this is a movement where the horse changes leads at the canter every stride—"and he would start getting internal again. I couldn't risk it. I didn't want him to get fried again." Instead Ruth eased up on Charmont, accepting that the current miracle was miracle enough. Now one of her students has Charmont as her schoolmaster. "The horse is working in his comfort zone," she says, "and he is clam-happy.

"The last thing about Charmont," Ruth says, "is that after I'd ridden a test, and it was good, I was holding Charmont and chatting with Dr. Soule"—Dr. Soule, her veterinarian, had always shared Ruth's conviction that the horse was salvageable—"and a man walked by while we were talking. Whoever this man was, he was maybe twenty feet away. And Charmont just flipped out—he reared up and screamed, pawing the air, and I just didn't know at all what was happening. Then the horse settled down, and I asked Dr. Soule, 'What was *that?*' And he said, 'Don't you know?' 'Know what?' 'That was the trainer who fractured this horse's leg six years ago while schooling canter pirouettes.'" Ruth pauses. "Six *years*," she says, quietly amazed.

The redemption of Charmont follows a story line that we all know by heart and never tire of—it offers heroes and villains and dramatic symmetry, and these are all things that people have powerful receptors for. Yet there is a counternarrative to redemption that pulls on the other arm, and it does not surprise me at all that Ruth also has one of these. Many experienced riders do.

In 1993, Ruth took in training a horse who had been hand-raised after being orphaned as a foal. This human foster parenting sounds sweet on the surface, and the beginning of a horse story that will end with affection and success, but the truth is that horses raised this way often have something missing. Horses need each other to convey social norms—how to dance, submit, sniff poop, follow directions, run from tigers; if they do not know these things, they often go funny in the head. Ruth knew his history and sensed his deficits: "He'd never been kicked around in a group of other horses, and he'd never been taught the basics, the business of respecting personal space and minding your manners, and of course everyone thought it was so cute when he was a foal that he'd rear up and put his feet on your shoulders. But it isn't cute. It's dangerous. The real problem was that he'd never taken Horse 101, and he didn't understand anything at all about boundaries. But I said okay, send him over, and we'll get him backed"—a term for introducing a young animal to being ridden—"and I guess I'd been on and riding him maybe six weeks, and things were going pretty well. But sometimes you just know about a horse, that they're mean or there's something wrong. You can feel it, and you can see it in their eyes.

"I had a strong feeling that this horse was going to stand up with me eventually, but every time I sensed he was thinking about it, I'd just change the subject—we'd change direction or canter or trot over a crossrail, do something to get him thinking about something else. This worked well for a while. So then one day we're cantering to the left, coming down the long side of the indoor school, and he just stopped. I legged him on and nothing happened, and I was carrying a little jumping bat and I tapped him on the shoulder. Not hard, just *tap*, and he stood straight up and backed me into the wall. I knew I was in big trouble, and I knew I had to get off, but I *couldn't* get off because the wall was behind me. I really don't remember how many times he did that, but eventually I was able to sort of scoot him away from the wall into the middle of the arena.

"I'd had a horse in the past who would rear and just walk the whole arena on his back legs, so it wasn't really the rearing itself that was worrying me—it was more my sense that this horse wasn't normal and he really wanted me gone. So I dropped my stirrups and started sliding off the back. My feet were just an inch or two off the ground, and that's when he bucked. And he didn't kick me because I was too close to him, but he *lifted* me, he sent me up in the air and forward, way over his head. I was flying, and the worst part was that I was up there so long that I had time to get my feet back under me, and so when I landed, more on my right foot than my left, I shot my tibia and fibia bone through my knee and my femur through my hip bone. Like a bullet. Everything just shattered."

We enter into our dealings with horses unarmed—we really can't do otherwise—but it can be an expensive transaction. Ruth, for example, couldn't ride for nearly a year, and the riding she could do at first was lopsided; some riders, perhaps even many riders, after an accident of this magnitude, do not have the commitment to come back. "Did you ever think you wouldn't?" I ask.

"No. No. I never thought that. I explained to the doctors that I was going to ride in the Olympics someday, and I was ready to do what I had to do to get there. 'Just tell me,' I said. 'I'll do it.' It took a long time, and not all of them believed I could do it, but I did. I'm very stubborn." But the sheer scope of this injury—bone fragments everywhere and massive structural damage—meant that Ruth, for a long time, needed something else to do. And at the risk of making it sound trivial, what Ruth did was go shopping.

"I went to Denmark to be with Bo"—then her fiancé and now her husband—"and the whole experience there was a good one. I learned Danish, and that was very useful. I even learned how to cook. And I figured that I couldn't ride but I could drive, so I began making friends and contacts, and I started looking at horses. That was the first time I ever brought horses over from Denmark—five, that first time, four for different students, and then Mastermind." Mastermind, with Ruth riding, was the American Horse Shows Association Horse of the Year at first level in 1994 and the U.S. Dressage Federation reserve champion at Intermediate in 2000. But she was not shopping at the top, at the equine equivalent of Fifth Avenue, since Ruth's interest lies in finding the affordable, average horse with willingness and spark. These horse-hunting trips are now a regular part of Ruth's calendar, although—oddly, it seems—Ruth does not talk much about her bargain hunter's eye or her intuition for matching horses to specific riders. Instead she says only that she has found a niche for herself: "Lots of people spend more money than they need to. I have a barn full of average horses, but they generally don't stay that way. With the right training, you can go a long way with an average horse."

I have to ask Ruth, as the interview winds down, whether she has ever gone into that riding trance where everything goes perfectly. "Yes," she says, instantly recognizing what I mean. "Those happen, and all you can say about it later was that it was beautiful. You kind of fall into it, it becomes this ball, this package, and it isn't about any individual movement but more a singsongy thing, and a pattern, and you feel like maybe you're watching yourself at a distance, and it's beautiful. You can't even talk about it. If you have a bad test, you can tell someone else every single thing that went wrong, but when you get a ride like that there's no single thing, it's all one thing, and the only thing to say about it is that it was beautiful."

Ruth pauses. "I'm not a golfer," she says, "and I'm not interested in golf. But one day a friend took me out to a driving range, and I could see right away how golf could be like dressage. I could hit the ball pretty well because I've learned how to concentrate, and because I could hit it this far, then next time I wanted to make this little adjustment and then hit it *that* far. And then I had to hit it again and fix this little thing to see what would happen with that. It became this mini obsession for me, and I began to see that this is how people get engaged, this is how they connect, this is how they indulge themselves in their sports. Because from the outside of golf, we don't see much—a bunch of people walking around on the grass—and people see us riding horses and it's probably the same thing. I think it probably looks pretty dull, just women on horses going around in circles. But the inside—the inside is the part that matters."

As I walk back to my car, I see that the barns are curiously empty—no 4-Hers loafing in the aisles, no boarders doing tack or stalls, no one in the indoor arena. It's odd, and it takes several long moments for me to finally compute that summer is over, school has started, and the standing army of young girls has been reassigned, at least until Saturday morning, to U.S. History and Algebra I. There are no voices, no mumbling radios. Horses doze and chew and make the hundred small noises large animals at rest like to make—they sigh, wuffle, fart, rub, and rattle their faces hopefully around inside their feed buckets. I see Reba, motionless and staring out the main entrance—her box stall is the one nearest the door—and by following her gaze I look across the sunlit yard to where a cat drinks studiously from a puddle. I then call on Prince, who stands foursquare, nodding vigorously and a little autistically, as if involved in complex conversation with an invisible friend. He's an utter mess—during his turnout he stumbled on a burr plantation, rubbed them all over his body, matted them, and even worked out how to make his mane clump into little fists of chocolate-colored hair and sticky balls of prickly vegetation. His forelock pops up like a deranged topiary; I can't see his tail in the shadows, and I probably don't want to. When I speak to him he breaks off his curious conversation with himself and puts his wiggly nose between the bars, takes my shirt between his teeth, and gives it an experimental pull. "Are you bored?" I ask him. He can't understand the question but knows enough to recognize it as an inquiry, and he answers by releasing my clothes and pressing his blocky yellow face against the bars. He looks silly, but I can't suppress a rush of complicated admiration. Prince is Prince, and he cares nothing for appearances. And Ruth is right—the inside really is the part that matters.

THIRTEEN

WHEN WE TELL OUR STORIES ABOUT HORSES, THEY ANSWER BY telling us the truth, which can make for an unsettling transaction. Even though all animals are generically honest—they can't be otherwise—they really do vary in how much they play along with the human urge to shape events into fiction. Dogs, for example, often accommodate us with great sensitivity, sometimes accepting a leading role in the family melodrama; most of us know of households where Fido is the object of endless and often quite uninteresting discussion. Even cats can contribute to the domestic narrative, though far more obliquely, but as we have seen these companion animals have a high level of indoorsy affection that horses simply do not have. This isn't an equine moral posture, but a result of simply being horses. Of course horses can be wrong in their truthfulness—they may report a tiger in the laundry basket or a brace of dragons flying overhead—but this wrongness isn't deception. Horses do not lie.

This leads to more problems than you'd think, mostly because we humans claim superior knowledge and access to the truth. To complicate matters, we are ourselves skilled and elaborate liars. It can be argued, cogently I think, that one of the big things that sets humans apart from other animals is our passion for dissembling. This passion goes by other, nicer names—metaphor, storytelling, mythmaking, poetics—but it often yanks us away from understanding plain animal utterances.

I learned this lesson the hard way from Bones. Because she fidgeted and had a lot of unwarranted opinions, I slid easily into the posture of the tolerant mother, which meant I often ignored any response I didn't approve of. This approach seemed humane and neutral and reflected well on me; it also meant, on some deeper and lazier level, that I had less static in my life, less information to process, and less to do. She would still sometimes twirl in the cross ties, bump me, rush ahead, lag behind, and make rude faces at me behind my back; once I got on, she was mostly obedient, but she always reserved the right to bounce up and down in one place and paw at the ground when I asked her to stand still. My planned ignoring of her outbursts was meant to be soothing and nonreinforcing, but it didn't work; she never got bored with her behavior, and it took me a long time to realize that there was something about it that was intrinsically gratifying. Every time she bumped me out of balance, every time I yielded, she was manufacturing her own reward. She would lift her head in triumph: *I win.*

But here's the thing: By this time she *was* winning, in at least two conflicting senses of the word, since during this same time she was also improving incrementally in her ring work, on the trails, and over fences. As I adapted, coaxed, ignored, and made allowances, I found I could now finesse her around a course of jumps at a local show and, because she was so talented, win a goodly share of prizes. I could even enter a hack class where, if there were no explosions, I could exploit her forwardness and her flashy style. Her coloring was decidedly unfashionable, but she was also impossible to miss among the bays and chestnuts. If a hack class has forty horses in it, it helps to be memorable.

This sounds like progress, and at the time it felt like progress, but it wasn't solid because it was partially grounded in deceit. By pretending that her attempts to dominate me didn't really matter, I was actually keeping the domination conversation alive. I wasn't really smart enough to know this, but, like the business with the bridle and the Necco wafer, I was smart enough to know when something bothered me, despite having other evidence—in this case, ribbons in various colors—that things were fine.

Then one spring I was allowed to move her temporarily to a local teaching barn where I could get more instruction and where, for the first time in her rather long life, she was expected to live in a box stall. She hated it, and deteriorated into pacing and sulking, and the obvious fix was to simply let her live outdoors again. She genuinely and absolutely preferred it—most horses do—and there happened to be a large turnout yard and shed behind the main barn where a dozen or so reliable school horses loafed and rolled and grimaced at each other in what appeared to be largely symbolic, recreational confrontations. So Bones, despite being a paying, box-stall boarder, was deposited into this good-natured, somewhat blue-collar neighborhood, which she organized with amazing speed and assurance into a tight, delinquent band of troublemakers. I was awestruck—she had always been the second-stringer at home, accepting instruction and correction from my sister's Standardbred, a horse blessed with deep reserves of poise and rectitude. Freed from Baby's tyranny, Bones became a thug. Within three days, she had all the horses taking cues from her, refusing to be caught, and moving as one across the half acre of grubby, broken ground. By the end of the week, she was in complete, undisputed charge of all hay piles, watering stations, and rules of proximity. No child could wander innocently into this equine Mafia to catch Spotty or Smoky or Bruce; no amount of gentle bribery could divide or conquer.

Bones's new criminal status was embarrassing and disruptive, but two good things came of it. First, I realized that my scatty, troubled mare was not the basket case I had always assumed her to be, and that I'd badly misjudged her. But second, I felt compelled to hang over the rail and watch as this herd went about its business, something I'd never had an opportunity to do before. Once I got accustomed to its swirly logic, I began to grasp that horse society is a profound matriarchy. I hadn't understood this before—I had a bunch of squishy, rather sexist ideas, derived mostly from horse stories, that stallions were somehow in charge of things. If no stallion was in the offing, I went on to assume, unthinkingly, that the geldings would be in charge.

Not true. I learned later that stallions are, quite literally, peripheral presences; a young stud horse in the wild will wander alone or in a bachelor group until a band of mares and their young offspring consent to his presence, provided he behaves. This last point is important, since, when it comes to mares, their standards are high and their decisions are final. Jane Smiley, that consummate observer of equine behavior, describes this dynamic in her novel *Horse Heaven*. A recently gelded, unusually aggressive specimen named Epic Steam has discovered that he can jump out of his isolated pasture and engage in an extended meet-and-greet with other horses on the farm. Eventually he finds himself "just where he wanted to be for so very long, in a paddock with four mares. Something this exciting for the four mares hadn't happened in years, so they stood stock-still, ears pricked, tails up, staring at him."

> He took this as encouragement, and lifted his own tail, arched his neck, and progressed in a beautiful *passage* around the perimeter of the pasture, picking his feet up as quick and high

as if the ground were strewn with hot coals. All the horses in every other pasture looked on and occasionally whinnied encouragement. After displaying himself to his own satisfaction, Epic Steam lowered his head and snaked it toward one of the mares, a little bay. He approached her. She moved away, toward the other mares, and he paused, but then approached again. Manners do not come naturally to a young stallion, and did not come naturally to Epic Steam in any event. Her retreat aroused some of his inherent aggression, and he went after her. He thought he might bite her. Intent upon this thought, he did not pay attention to his position relative to the other mares, and so he did not realize until it was already happening that they were kicking the stuffing out of him.

The reader cheers—this particular horse has been in need of a comeuppance for some time now—but the deeper point is that this scene is a counternarrative to the established tale of the proud, wily stallion who dominates his mares and assumes the role of chief executive. This alternate version isn't feminism run amok; it actually happens to be true. An alpha mare is a formidable and profoundly social creature, and leaning over the fence watching Bones run everything I began to understand that her endless bumps and challenges, her squirminess, and her willingness to crowd me was something I should no longer deceive myself about or studiously ignore. She would not stop out of boredom, because it didn't bore her; instead it was primal and compelling. And hard to bring to closure—it took two skilled handlers most of an afternoon to settle the herd, siphon off the school horses, catch her, and then seduce her back into her old dominance pattern with me, which must have seemed pretty insipid after seven days of the real thing.

It was only after this encounter that I began to develop an enduring love for watching horses in groups at liberty, since this is when they wear their truthfulness—their wishes and decisions—on their metaphorical sleeves. At East Hill, where horses are turned out with an almost obsessive regularity, in all but the most horrible weather, the opportunities to do this are ongoing—horse society there is allowed to operate in clusters of twos and threes, and even the unredeemably rowdy ones, who really have to be kept by themselves, still have an opportunity to gossip over the fence. This is healthy, even though it means the animals are often dirty; I have visited and briefly worked in barns where the horses were almost never at liberty, and they spent most of their time spanking clean but going quietly (or not so quietly) insane.

All this fence hanging has taught me that what often matters to a horse is something as basic as whether he can get another horse to move. Like the talent for mapping, this is essentially a spatial behavior, and space, for horses, is packed with meaning. Where they are, where they stand in relationship to each other, what they do about it, and what happened when all were assembled here the last time are the important social verbs that drive what will happen now; *now* is the construct that horses pay attention to, and it sometimes seems that their prodigious and detailed memories do not really exist for learning or reflection, but for refining and animating *now*. As a group of horses moves out to grass, in for feeding, or from one place in the pasture to another, they act out complex little dramas about leading, following, clustering, and standing ground, and the results of these transactions are often surprising. The best horse in the barn—well schooled, fun to be around, responsive, and even-tempered—is hardly ever the best horse in equine society, which is perhaps more proof that horses and people do not really agree on what's important.

With Bones back home in the pasture with Baby, I was able to see something that hadn't registered before. Baby, unlike my big spotted mare, was never thuggish or punishing—watching them together, all I could see was equilibrium. They grazed close together and spent huge amounts of time doing what looked like nothing at all. Horses can be spectacularly idle, and the two of them loafed, scratched, swished away flies, snoozed, watched the wildlife, and made leisurely strolls of the perimeter. Every now and again, they would buck and play. If we needed to rotate the two of them from one pasture to another—a very common exercise in my foster mother's grazing program—we would set the gates, pick up the water buckets, call to Baby, and the two of them would trot complacently up or down the long driveway, technically loose but completely under control. Baby came when she was called, and Bones followed Baby.

The vast difference between this arrangement and the quarreling I had witnessed at the other barn was more than a little confusing, and it took me a while to find a name for what I was seeing. This wasn't just the absence of discord; it seemed obvious that these two were friends. But *friendship* is a tricky term. Many of the people who study animals—including the primatologists who study our very closest relatives—sometimes call friendship *the f-word*, because it's been so folded and smudged by human fingers. It's hard to know, they say, what really goes on between two animals of the same species who hang around together. These creatures may not be, in the sense we mean, actual friends, although I have to add that this objection seems a little fussy, since there's no question that many animals form social bonds that have nothing to do with reproduction or kinship or advancing their DNA. Why should we assume that, when humans do it, it's somehow different and needs a distinctive name? It is also hard not to notice that these supposedly nonessential relationships are the very thing that makes both animals and people more interesting. Recreational bonds, whether we call them friendships or not, are well worth watching, and it was by watching that I learned that Baby was the undisputed alpha horse because she was completely sure of herself and utterly trustworthy, and Bones put faith in her in exactly the way I yearned for her to put faith in me. They were at peace together, a kind of equine binary star.

This trustworthiness, this final confidence, is what riders like Ruth have and I do not. My greatest flaw as a rider, then and now, is that I am not always sure I know what I want to have happen. I'm not talking here about navigational things—I can almost always get to the jump, around the barrel, through the gate, across the pasture, or up the hill. But there are other things, subtler things—*dressage* things—and these are what really matter. There's a way to travel and a way not to, and the difference has to do with intangibles like style and forwardness and way of going—these terms refer to the horse's physical state and level of happiness with the proceedings, and mainly tell us that riding is more than the mere fact of arrival.

These important intangibles have always eluded me. I know when things are going badly, but I have no clear picture in my mind of how I want them to go, and this has tended to make me tentative and blank and hopeful. This absence of mental aggression is what makes it hard for me to succeed with a horse like Railund, who relies absolutely on having a definite, controlling, rather bossy rider. But the upside to being vague is that horses with ideas—Abbott, Prince, Reba—would often fill up that blank space with their own material, and this gave me access to the very thing that attracted me to riding in the first place. I wanted to know, feel, and be able to think about horses in a firsthand way; I liked it when they did this, since it was a way for them to be present and truthful with me.

The trouble with the truth is that it can be unattractive and uncomfortable—there were times, on Bones, when I felt like I was on a trampoline, and other times when I felt caught in a blender. This wasn't just bad behavior, and I want to digress for a moment and say that the word *just* should be stricken forever from a rider's vocabulary: "He's just being a stinker," "He's just trying to scare me," "He's just not listening," are all sentences that dismiss the thing that matters with horses, which is *now*. By using this word, we lapse into telling ourselves a story that we hope will turn out differently tomorrow, which is a thing a horse never thinks about. One thing I continually appreciate about Kathie's teaching is that I never hear this word. She sometimes says a problem *doesn't matter*, but I think she means something different by this—when Prince drops unexpectedly out of his canter into a scrambling trot, or when Reba's backlog of awkwardness catches up with her, she uses this phrase to indicate that, *now* notwithstanding, it is not possible to do everything at once.

The problem of *now* certainly applied to my dominance struggle with the spotted mare—after the episode with the school horses, I saw for the first time that her boorishness wasn't just bad behavior. She, like Epic Steam, could be a monumental troublemaker, and her need to win had more momentum than my need for a reasonable level of tranquillity. I also saw that if I entered into a direct war with her on the issue, she would love every minute of it, and she would also, most assuredly, defeat me—horses are very strong. All I really had on my side of the ledger was that she had already made many important concessions, that we had come to know and understand each other, and so something was at stake for both of us. Thinking about Baby, and about friendship, I concluded that it was my job to become not just a rider she mostly consented to carry, but a rider who was somehow trustworthy.

So I began riding her alone. This was fairly new for both of us—except for the occasional schooling session in the ring, we tended, generally, to ride out in company of twos or threes, and sometimes as part of a congenial larger lump of other horses. Baby was almost always there, a soothing presence, and this happy scrum also meant the humans could chatter, making it a social event for everyone. But I decided that, for me to become trustworthy, Bones and I had to spend more time out in the woods and fields together.

This decision made her horribly anxious, and when she was anxious she became noisy, shouting and weeping as she stomped through the woods, calling out endlessly for an acceptable companion. Her old reactiveness returned; there were tigers everywhere; when I finally turned her back toward the stable, she leaned into my hands, jigging and flailing in frustration that she couldn't go faster. I became so accustomed to the lift and shiver of the saddle as she whinnied that I hardly paid attention, although the decibel level did embarrass me—as we thrashed our way down the trails and dirt roads around town, people stepped out on their porches to see what all the noise was about and perhaps to check up on me. I don't blame them—it sounded as if I were extracting her teeth with rusty pliers. Bones would roll up into a tight, unhappy ball, bounce, squall, dribble, crimp her tail, and periodically vent her upset with a potent outburst of bucking. With her rolling eyes, her noise, and her splashy coloration, I think we made quite a spectacle, escapees from some demonic merry-go-round.

It wasn't much fun, but it sort of worked. With only me to fall back on, my mare discovered that her isolation really wasn't absolute: I spoke, I made decisions, I directed her as best I could, and she always managed to come home uneaten, despite the many tigers. She realized she wasn't going to die gradually, over the course of about a month—a difficult month, but one well worth getting through. She didn't like this forced acceptance very much, but still gradually toned down the racket and even, at times, seemed to acquiesce without resentment, cocking her ears back toward me as I chose the safe route around the unacceptable puddle. Like with the business with the halter, *hup*, and *ho*, the ground between us shifted again, and again to my slight advantage. But I found the state of things coercive and disagreeable.

Then my older brother, Allan, went to the pound and got a dog. This was a background, household sort of event, done on an impulse that didn't involve me, although I liked the dog. His name was Ranger—a good name for a dog-pound animal—and he looked like a cross between some sort of husky and some sort of generic, big-headed hound. He had impenetrable fur that was layered and curiously short, a soaring and distinctive *olla-olla* call, and more skin than a dog his size was really entitled to. Despite his iffy, jailbird background, Ranger was free of any kennel neurosis and went at life with a healthy doggy vigor: He swam, hunted, womanized, and carried disgraceful and smelly things around in his mouth, but above all these things nothing made him happier than an expedition. This is how, within a week or two of his arrival, Ranger became the third leg of a weird and unplanned three-legged stool, since he would not let me go out for a ride without him.

Relations between species are hard to categorize, and it's important not to romanticize or misjudge what happens. This is especially the case when we talk about domestic animals, where our urge to make up a story can be almost irresistible. So I must be careful here, and simply tell what I think must be the truth, which is that Bones, at least some of the time, did not particularly care about Ranger, and Ranger, for his part, was probably more interested in horse excrement than he was in horses themselves. Yet there he was, a sudden presence in our daily doings, and his bumptious and smiling being radically transformed the proceedings.

Dogs like to go scouting. Nothing pleases them more than the sort of outing where they are free to circle forward, let you slide by, cross you to leeward, and appear magically in the lead again—and Ranger took scouting to heart. As far as he was concerned, the entire point of existence was to secure the moving perimeter and verify that the landscape was operating smoothly, and, in an unusual intersection of desires, this was a task that my mare desperately wanted performed. Whatever residual worries she had about my ability to protect her simply vanished, and there is no question that they vanished only when Ranger was there.

I agreed with Bones that Ranger was an excellent escort, and I got a huge amount of pleasure out of watching him do his job. While we stuck to the trail, he would break ground out ahead of us in a kind of huge fan, crossing and recrossing our line of travel, the white tip of his tail mostly visible above the scrubby undergrowth. He would then fall backward or off to the side to inspect holes, wet places, and evidence of animal life, and this sometimes involved the unexpected appearance of a rabbit or pheasant. Bones was interested in and sometimes startled by these animal materializations, but they didn't seem to actually frighten her. Ranger would then fall behind—sometimes far behind—and when this happened he would race to catch up, his tongue hanging sideways and his expression at once joyful and businesslike. He then began the entire scouting pattern all over again—he crashed ahead of us through the bushes, plunged into streams, and generally made an amazing racket, all of which my horse monitored with interest. Sometimes he would gallop right up on her heels—a fine excuse for an explosion—and she merely noted his return with satisfaction and composure. When we reached an open place—a cornfield or the local tree nursery with its potbellied arborvitae standing in unnatural rows—Ranger made a point of closing ranks and circling us rather tightly, and more than once he nearly tangled himself under the mare's hard, pumping feet. She hopped to avoid stepping on him, he scooted, and we all continued on as if nothing exciting had happened, which it obviously hadn't.

Ranger brought to these long rides the confidence and knowledge that I lacked, since he obviously understood that tigers were out there and was determined to find and vanquish them. The result was that Bones traveled happily on a long rein, swinging her neck and back, and was perfectly fine about standing still while I checked my bearings or drank some water. She went uphill and down, into thick places and dark places and narrow places and queer places; she even stepped daintily through the puddles she'd once assumed to be a mile deep and requiring a prolonged detour. Better still, she stopped bumping and crowding, and, for the first time, began showing me some signs of routine affection—she ran her wiggly nose over my chest and neck when I brushed her face and sighed with pleasure when I rubbed stinky, soothing liniment on her hardworking legs. The transformation was quick, and quite impressive.

I have a photograph of our triumvirate, Ranger in the foreground and horse and handler in the midground, that captures this odd arrangement. It must have been taken in either late fall or early spring, since I am cooling my horse with a rug thrown over her haunches and the front folded back and buckled over her withers so her chest is exposed. Her winter coat is either growing in or shedding out—it's impossible to tell which—and the trees along the driveway look chilled and bare. A trick of elevation—I am walking on the high mound in the middle of road, while Bones is walking on the low dip made by passing tires—makes me look even taller than I actually am; my horse looks curiously medium-sized, as opposed to the very substantial horse she really was. Horse, dog, and human are all tired, damp, and dirty; Bones walks next to me, her shoulder exactly level with mine, her head lowered and her ears tuned backward toward me. She curls her head and neck around me very slightly, interested in my agenda, but her weather eye is glued on Ranger, who, even so close to home, is still taking his job seriously and breaking trail. Everything about her body language signals contentment, willingness, submission; everything about mine conveys a disheveled, unthinking happiness. My braids are coming loose, my hands are in my pockets, and I do not see a lead rope anywhere. Yet we are deeply tethered, the three of us, by a common, treasured enterprise. When I look at this picture, which I do often because it sits on my desk, I understand it captures a moment of peace and equilibrium. In it, I seem to loom over the horse who once dominated me, and who now chooses to walk freely and respectfully in my orbit. For my part, I am built around a smile, and the message in that smile is plain: *I win.*

FOURTEEN

WITHOUT PREAMBLE AUTUMN ARRIVES, AND REBA IS BEGINNING to put on weight. She has always been a little thin, a little weedy looking; now it's noticeable that her chest and neck are starting to bulk up a little. Most of this is muscle—her stringy outline is slowly being upgraded with new, subtle upholstery—but some of it is extra Reba, so that she looks, for the first time, like a horse with something in reserve. The sharp, thin air, combined with her improving condition, makes her quicker and more determined, so that some days she leans hard on the bit, especially on the right side, blistering my ring finger since I don't like riding in gloves and don't ride well enough to persuade her to stop. Other days she insistently volunteers slow, hard, focused bouts of cantering, very different from her previous skittering. She seems to be getting something out of her system with this three-beat, utterly steady expenditure of her new excess calories, and I can feel through the saddle that the longer she canters, the clearer her mind is. We both welcome these long, hypnotizing waltzes, although they are sometimes difficult to bring to an end—whatever hard question she is turning over in her mind seems to require almost endless kinetic processing.

By midfall, I realize I am beginning to love her. This is not the brief infatuation I had for the unhappy Dr. Denton, but something far more complicated and responsible. I want Reba to become progressively more exactly like herself, more expressive, and this desire is clean, free of dreams of personal glory. This love is also unrequited, since Reba is not really very interested in me. Unlike Prince, she does not seem to know me from Adam, although her attachment to Kathie is obvious. As happens with love, her indifference only fuels my desire for her presence. I think about her often, and especially in the early mornings as I get ready to go to work, and during the long drive to Burlington I strategize over her welfare. I am worried about her endless lugging on my right hand—a thick blistered sore, on its way to becoming a callus, has erupted on the side of my ring finger, and this gets picked at throughout the day, the skin shedding in papery strips around a hard pink oval. I decide I want to try her in a different bit, one that she might be less likely to lean against, and one dark morning, still wet from the shower, I find myself digging around in my old tack trunk, looking for the French-link snaffle I used on a Thoroughbred I bought as a yearling and had for a couple of years before a divorce meant giving her up. I like these bits, and seem to have two of them. They have loose, triple-jointed mouthpieces, very smooth, with an appealing thickness, and I remember that the filly, a stubborn but sensible horse named Rose, found them chewable and kind and surprisingly difficult to grab on to—something about their yielding architecture and loose play made them hard to grip. I put them in my car to show to Kathie, but the next time I am at the barn I see that Kathie, as always, is ahead of me: Reba's old full-cheek Fulmer bit has been substituted with a triple-jointed snaffle almost identical to my own. I like that we think the same, but feel slightly thwarted—I want to give Reba something that is mine.

A cold, sunny autumn brings with it a near hysteria in the maple trees, and the color is perhaps too intense for ordinary eyes. The tunnels of forest are a screaming red—it's beautiful but disconcerting, as if the trees are in genuine turmoil. My nose runs, the nights are dry and biting, and Vince and I huddle sadly around the stove, unready for the end of what has proved to be a damp and luminous summer. Each day is darker and more abbreviated; time feels short, precious, and paralyzing. The pumpkins for sale at the farm stand have hot, perfect skin and a glandular tightness that makes it impossible to decide which specimen to buy, and it is while sorting through these orange globes, unable to choose, that I realize that part of the problem is that the thing I really want to buy is Reba. I want to own her life, claim her, and see what happens next. As Tolstoy's Strider has already observed, however, this is a perverse urge, to say nothing of expensive. I finally pick two fat, fluorescent pumpkins, but their satisfying heft does little to dampen my acquisitiveness. Just thinking about Reba, which I do too much, makes me ache with greed.

My finances will not let me own a horse, but a systems check reveals that, if I give up my swimming-pool membership, I could ride more often. I like this idea, and Kathie and I figure out how to slide in another session every week, this one with another adult rider who is better than me but not ridiculously so. These new arrangements are patted into place on the same sharp, windy morning that Reba royally dumps me, a thing she executes with precision and skill. It's impossible for me to sort out what actually happens: We are trotting to warm up, and then several new things happen at once, and then I am springing up from the ground to catch her. I am surprised and unhurt, and some part of me enjoys it—there is something competent and casual about the way it unfolds, as if

Reba were a champion chess player up against an unworthy opponent. She does, technically, buck, but I feel more as if I've been shrugged or flicked away.

I put Reba on the longe line—standard procedure after an infraction like this one—and she surprises both me and Kathie by offering up a truly impressive array of delinquent behavior, bucking, skidding, racing, farting, and prancing with her head high in the air. It's an amazing outburst for such a studious and careful animal. Each time she starts to settle down, she suddenly remembers—*I'm bad now!*—and begins again. It strikes me as a little melodramatic, although the underlying angst is undoubtedly authentic. Because I love her, it's easy to be patient and let her vent. Still, when she finally signals she is ready to behave, I make rather a point of sending her on for longer than she is entirely happy with. Finally, wet and winded, she moves her feet simply because I want her to, and canters slowly and sadly in a resigned, symmetrical circle. I decide it is time to climb aboard again.

"You're brave," says Kathie, and the way she says this tells me that the fall looked far worse than it was. I don't know how to tell Kathie that I want to own this mare, and want to even more now that I know how easily she can get rid of me. For some reason, this new information about her doesn't frighten me at all—it mostly reminds me that sometimes the tigers of wrath really are wiser than the horses of instruction. The poet William Blake said that in a collection of impenetrable announcements he called *The Marriage of Heaven and Hell*, and what seemed to interest Blake while he wrote it were the ideas of freedom, movement, and the virtues of velocity. "Expect poison," he tells us, "from the standing water." Blake was probably a little nuts, but eerily right in at least some of his particulars; for him, the mute imperative of living is pried loose from life's unpleasant consequences. "The cut worm," he says, "forgives the plow." What's more, I am now forcefully reminded that Reba, like all horses, has to balance the demands of many wrathful tigers, and even though I do not like being dumped, and I am certainly too old to be dumped often, I like and understand the style of her choosing.

We go back out onto the track, I give her a few minutes to catch her breath, and we resume the lesson. Reba trots and canters wisely, cautiously, submissively, and I talk to her a little more than usual. *Good girl*, I say. *Good girl.* When I strip off her saddle and clean her up, I am surprised and a little gratified to see that she is finally noticing me, and I dawdle shamelessly, carefully fluffing up the matted wet places around her ears, grooming her underbelly, brushing her silky tail, and rubbing all four legs with a luxurious quantity of liniment. She tracks my movements with her ears and from the corners of her unusual eyes—the strange bare patches around these eyes have started to grow in white, so it's a little like being scrutinized by a clown fish or perhaps that dog in the Target commercials. About halfway through this long process, she heaves an enormous sigh. This is a good sound; it means, unambiguously, that she has let go of something that was worrying her.

The approaching cold brings another abrupt disturbance: Railund is suddenly dead, taken by a bout of colic. He had been out at a sales barn for a while, being looked at by potential buyers, and his disappearance and eventual return was simply part of the tidal quality of any large horse barn—animals drift in and out of the picture plane in a way that can be hard for an erratic visitor like me to really follow. One day he got on the trailer; on some different day he came off it again, unpurchased but apparently none the worse for wear. Then suddenly he announced his discomfort, went down, sweated, thrashed with pain, and never got up again. I know these things can happen, but the terrible dull truth of it frightens me, in part because he always seemed utterly indestructible. There is sorrow in the barn, tinged with guilt, although his sickness progressed so rapidly that the vet could do nothing. I try to reconcile this loss with his big trot and his reliable charity, but the dots do not connect.

Colic is a result of the fragile equine digestive system, which is explicitly designed to process a steady supply of rough forage, consumed in small quantities pretty much all the time. In the wild, horses eat for many hours at a stretch, snooze or conduct social business for a while, and then eat for several hours more; often this grazing is poor and scrubby. To compensate, free horses will experiment with other chewable things—bushes, buds, twigs, bark, thistles, fruit, acorns, and almost any other item that for some reason looks appealing. This sounds indiscriminate, but horses are actually surprisingly skilled, fussy eaters; they rarely consume anything toxic, and judge plants speedily and accurately by taste and smell. One reason the upper lip of a horse is so expressive, wriggly, and prehensile is that it is used to sort plants by their feel and odor, and to push untasty or poisonous plants out of the way.

Sadly, most domesticated horses do not feed this way. In the United States, most barns begin the morning with a round of hay, a seemly pause, and a ration of processed grain. This is often followed by hay in the middle part of the day, hay in the late afternoon, and a second ration of grain, bulked up with hay, in the early evening. Water is present all the time, and in general the quality of this feed is high, but this diet is both more monotonous and more discrete than the equine body is really set up for. We may think four meals a day would be quite enough, but the horse is designed for a single lifelong meal that never really comes to what might be described as an end.

Added to this is a good deal of variation in what people think is proper food for horses, and in this matter the horses play along—

even the biggest equine fussbudget will tend to be adventurous in what he will consider eating. In the Middle East, horses are routinely offered table scraps, including meat, and in England I saw horses eat raw potatoes, gorse, and mangoes—this last item consumed with much rolling, squishing, and thumping, a general racket that I think I interpreted correctly as glee. Icelandic ponies thrive on fish and seaweed; Tibetan ponies eat sheep's blood mixed with grains; I once rode briefly at a barn where the horses were fed almost exclusively on stale, remaindered doughnuts, brought in by the truckload from a nearby bakery. An older but still respected veterinary text on my bookshelf says that a horse with a poor appetite can be offered "a couple of quarts of stout, ale, or porter, or a half a bottle of wine daily." Granted, the first edition of this text was printed in 1877, but this particular recommendation was still in there in 1972.

One upshot of these various human ideas about horse feeding can be colic, which is painful and dangerous. Horses can't puke, so if something suddenly disagrees with them they can't get rid of it quickly out the front end—the only way *out* is *through*. Which brings us to a second problem: The equine digestive system is delicately balanced. The stomach itself is relatively small, with a capacity of maybe a couple of gallons, and this is followed by large, surprisingly mobile intestines that are inordinately puckered, full of interstices, and easily blocked and twisted. Once this blockage or twisting happens, often as a result of rolling to relieve gassy discomfort, the end is nigh; a quick surgical intervention can sometimes yank the festering rabbit out of the hat, but not always. Railund, I learn after the fact, had already had one colic surgery like this, and a postmortem showed that he'd actually been building up to this episode for some time—there was evidence of necrosis in his digestive tract. Railund, a stoic personality, apparently never mentioned his discomfort to anybody, although it seems plausible to me that he might have tried at the other barn, with his complaints misinterpreted. If you don't know a horse well, his un-happiness is easy to dismiss: "He's just being a stinker"; "He's just trying to scare me"; "He's just not listening." Jeanette tells me about Railund's death, and the upsetting evidence from the post-mortem, with a kind of wondering grief; her theory, her story about it, is that Railund may have been toughing it out, waiting until he got home to die.

This is a difficult idea to evaluate. Horses know a lot about home, can always find their way back to it, and understand it to be special and safe. Yet I have to wonder whether a horse can stave off a fatal illness through a sheer act of will. What does seem possible is that Railund was offered a different diet in the other barn—rolled oats instead of sweet feed, sugar beet instead of bran—which may have brought on a subacute condition. He may have looked at his sides, or gotten nippy, or kicked grumpily at his stom-ach when his girth was tightened, but I am sorry to report that these are all normal, tiresome behaviors in the many, many horses that do not happen to be Railund. He may have been talking, but was unable to frame his message in a way that could be understood by strangers. It is this disturbing possibility that gives Jeanette's theory its potency; like Beauty's homecoming, it seems like a sen-timental pearl around a hard grain of truth. I think about it and find I want to cling to it despite my doubts, mostly because colic is so horrible, and he did nothing to earn a death like that.

I was well into early adulthood before colic became something more than a thing to read about, and I now know that this was not really luck. My foster mother—a dairy farmer, landscape architect, and horsewoman—kept our animals in managed grazing at least seven months out of the year. The pastures, which were not large but were very numerous, were tended, evaluated, reseeded, mowed, fertilized, scouted, rested, rotated, and obsessed over in a way that I did not then understand or appreciate. I did not even know enough to think it strange that we could work our animals quite hard four or five days a week on nothing but pasture, and that even at the height of fitness they all tended, if anything, to be rather plump; when the horses finally came in for good at the start of winter, they lived in a yard with a snug, south-facing loafing shed, where they spent a good portion of their time chewing their way steadily through what seemed like mountains of good-quality hay. We did not feed much grain—or potatoes, or fish blood, or wine—although we did keep some horse pellets and molasses around so we could persuade our horses to consume various medicines that were too icky to be eaten out of our hands. It wasn't until I left the home farm that I realized this was not the usual way of keeping horses; it also wasn't until I left that I saw colic, and how much it hurts, and how quickly it kills.

Yet Railund's death also reminds me of a home truth about horses, which is that anything can happen. A favorite weanling, straight-limbed and frisky and full of self-regard, can shatter a knee on a dip in the driveway; an experienced and sensible brood mare can die suddenly in childbirth; a reliable school horse can go mysteriously tippy, lopsided, and unwilling to move, a victim of a bug-borne neurological disease. These are the fatal cases. But horses can also break down unexpectedly, and not always from poor human judgment or from being given too much work to do. A minor flaw in soundness or conformation can trigger a cascade of problems that become progressively more unwieldy; an invisible genetic predisposition can lead to tumors, joint disease, skin cancer, blindness. Even with basically healthy horses, there is always something—wounds, bruises, scrapes, sore teeth, loose shoes, coughs, colds, swellings— and ownership is a gamble of both money and the heart. It seems that every horse offers a large and tempting target for tragedy.

I understand this dynamic because, on January 15, 1984, when Bones was thirty, my sister Caroline tacked her up and went for a routine winter constitutional around the large pond next to our house. Thirty is quite old for a horse, but this was no reason to avoid her allotment of exercise—except for a little spavin in her hind end from many years of cross-country work (all my fault), there was nothing about her physical condition that was even remotely worrisome, and she was accustomed to a prolonged quiet hack at least one day a week.

It was cold that day, about twelve degrees, and even though the snow cover wasn't thick, there were places where it had gone icy. The mare always wore spiked shoes in winter—they went on at about the same time the winter tires were mounted on the cars—but despite this precaution, despite her athleticism, despite her general fitness, there was one small, bad, and very specific moment when she lost her footing and tumbled down the steep shoreline, shedding an unhurt Caroline along the way. When eleven hundred pounds of spotted horseflesh reached the bottom of the embankment, her weight broke through the thin ice near the edge of the water and she suddenly found herself mired in the cold mud, branches, and tangle along the shoreline. She tried to get out of this mess but couldn't; Caroline later told me that, after her first big effort, her commitment to getting herself free suddenly eroded, and her struggles, if that's the right word, were curiously insipid for so energetic a horse. "It was as if a curtain had come down," she said. "It may have been the cold water, or it may have been something else, but she was in terrible trouble and she didn't seem to care." Caroline, always reliable in an emergency, headed back toward the house, yelling, and she simply kept on yelling until our father heard her and rescue operations began.

I wasn't there, and my mother, through the events that followed, made a strategic decision not to summon me—a good one, since I was pregnant and would probably have waded in, endangered my child, gotten frostbite, lost my composure, and generally added a high note of horror and upset to the proceedings. Instead, my mother called the fire department, the vet, and the neighbors; somewhere along the way the dog officer, the local police, and an ambulance all showed up for good measure. If I have counted correctly, at least eleven people and perhaps more converged on the woody shores of the pond to see if anything could be done about an old horse who had fallen through the ice.

I have a news clipping from the local paper about this accident. It says that when the rescue crew arrived, they found my mare "about ten feet from the shoreline, lying on its side in the mud. The owner [my foster father] was holding its head up to prevent it from drowning." I imagine this last detail with a mixture of admiration and profound anxiety—my foster father was then in his late sixties, and he had no business holding a horse's head out of the water of a frozen pond in the middle of January. He liked my horse well enough, even though he thought her hysterical and stupid, but it wasn't until that day that I realized how much he valued her. Whatever her shortcomings, I don't think he wanted her to die that way.

The firemen went into action without delay: They put a long rope around her middle and began pulling her out of the muck and ice toward the embankment. "For at least an hour, we pulled him closer and closer to the shoreline," Fire Captain Richard Goddard said—throughout the news clip, he never got her gender right, but it hardly matters. "It wasn't easy," he went on. "It was very cold, and there were so many sticks and branches and things that had to be cleared away." When Bones was finally close enough to the shore, they stopped pulling to see if she could get out on her own, but each time she tried she fell backward into the black hole of the open water again. This happened three times; after the last attempt, it was hard not to notice that Bones had now been struggling in the cold water for two hours, that she was growing increasingly listless, and that the rescue crew was running out of time.

It's unclear who decided what to do next—the story in the paper is murky on this point, and nobody I could ask specifically remembered—but it was abundantly clear by now that Bones was fading fast and could not climb out by the shoreline. I do know that it was Will Winchell, a neighbor, who borrowed the town fire truck, with all its heavy winches and come-alongs, and drove it carefully through the trees to a spot about a hundred feet down the shoreline. The idea, now, was to try to take my horse away from the steep embankment, out into the middle of the pond where the ice was thicker: Ice is slippery, but it does have the advantage of being flat. While Will secured the truck to several trees to keep it from slipping, someone produced a large square of old carpeting to lay over the sharp edge of the hole; someone else wrapped the old mare with complicated care in ropes and fire hoses. Then Will played out the fire truck's steel cable, ran across the ice, and hooked the ropes and hoses to the truck's four-ton winch. Somebody gave the signal, and the ominously still body of my spotted horse was slowly skidded up, out of the water, onto the carpet, and across about fifty feet of ice, where she lay, shrouded in restraints, on her left side. The vet gave her a shot of something—perhaps adrenaline or a painkiller—and insisted that the dripping, hypothermic mare be allowed to rest for a while. Then the vet and my mother took off the ropes and hoses to see what, if anything, was going to happen next. It seemed nearly impossible that anything could happen, since she'd gone into the water at 1:30 P.M. and it was now nearly dusk. People gathered to watch and, to everyone's genuine surprise, Bones propped on her chest, surveyed the proceedings, dug her cleated shoes into the ice, and stood. She walked off the pond, in the words of the fire captain, "as if nothing had happened." She wasn't even limping.

"That," my mother told the reporter, "was a miracle."

It was. This is a horse story that could easily have ended very differently, but that is not really the important thing about it, since it is mostly a story that illustrates how anything can happen around horses and eventually does. Where there are horses there are always surprises, and this contingent quality is always difficult to convey to people who have not stepped inside this universe, looked around, and decided to stay. A young, confident horse like Railund goes down, and an old, fretful one like Bones stands up, and there is no why. Uncertainty is a cost of doing business. In my twenties and early thirties, when I was teaching, I often felt uncomfortable and inadequate when I was asked what sounded like perfectly reasonable questions—*Will Ann do well at the show next weekend? How long before she will be able to jump?*—because I was already sensitized to the dangers of a firm answer. I always connected these queries to my early, mechanistic ideas about *correctness*, in that they assumed a horse world that was governed, at least on some level, by a set of rules. And perhaps it is, but they are not our rules. *Will the old horse come safely out of the frozen pond?* The only answer that suffices, I think, is *It all depends*.

Depends on what?

Beats me.

FIFTEEN

REBA HAS BEEN OUT IN A PADDOCK IN THE SEASON'S FIRST legitimate snow and now waits in the cross ties with ice on her whiskers. Since her delinquent episode, she has made several subtle changes, the most noticeable being that she no longer mutters while I groom her—she's relinquished the lippy, ongoing gestures of submissiveness that were once her primary way of appeasing her various tigers. These funny mouths are generally a good thing to see, since they indicate that the horse is in no mood for an argument, but in Reba their absence strikes me as an improvement. She seems to be signaling a new composure, and as part of the same shift in attitude she has also stopped making her grumpy face when I lift the saddle and put it on her back. She nods a little—residual anxiety—but the whole getting-ready transaction seems to have become less fraught, less demanding of her attention and mine.

This is not my doing. I can feel each time I ride her the progress that Kathie has made: Reba's body carriage, her whole feel, has become rounder, freer, and less awkward. Her less-good direction, to the left, no longer feels quite so choppy or insecure, and she has stopped collapsing and hanging on my outside hand; the hard lump on my finger has slowly receded. Better still, her steady one-two-one-two trot around the indoor arena now has a little swing in it, a small, bright bounce from behind, that has a prettiness I cannot see but know from Kathie's instruction must be there. I am still told to quiet my aids, sit deeper, ask for more power, and fix my somewhat sloppy position, but there are long moments when Kathie says nothing at all and only breaks the silence to say, "That's right. Now you've got her. Keep it going."

Sometimes I do see Reba's new prettiness, since Kathie will occasionally school her for a few minutes before I get on. I doubt if there is anything more absorbing than seeing a horse you covet get ridden, especially by someone who rides very well. Kathie is a small woman, and Reba is only a medium-sized horse, but the effect of the two of them together is striking since Reba, under Kathie, looks much bigger than she actually is. This change in proportion actually magnifies the progress that is being made: Reba, in the process of growing four or five imaginary inches, takes on a certain big-horse elegance. While still moving in a long frame, she can no longer be described as flat—her neck has a slight but becoming curve, and her back legs lift from the ground and reach beneath her. Her concentration is obvious—her ears are nearly motionless and convey the absolute focus that is the hallmark of everything that is Reba. Kathie slowly unlocks her neck and jaw, turning her head first one way and then another, before they step into a medium trot. They get comfortable and adjusted with each other, circling and changing direction, and then turn early out of the corner, about ten feet from the wall. There are a couple of strides of straightness, and then together they increase the flexion and quietly slide back to the wall again. Reba crosses her legs to make this sideways movement, and, as she does, there is a long moment of balletic grace that is both feminine and big—Reba's response to this movement is to blossom into a wider, more delicate animal. I can see her shoulders open; I can see the precise lightness of her feet on the springy tan-bark; I can even see her lift a little higher off the ground. This is the whole point of the exercise, called a leg yield. I have seen other people ride this movement with more polished outcomes, but Reba's rendition moves me with its honesty.

I generally do not get these kinds of results from Reba, but I do get a little more than I deserve, since the mare seems to have made a decision. In the two short weeks since her explosion, she has crossed a boundary, and she is no longer a half-schooled equine generalist but a legitimate, if low-level, dressage horse. I know this to be true not because she can do a good-enough leg yield, but because the heart of dressage, its final point, is simply to make a horse more beautiful. All the borrowed dressage words—*pirouette, half-pass, passage*—are not used to be fancy but to be precise and affectionate. They are words pressed into service because this kind of beauty is so hard to talk about. Watching the mare dance through another leg yield in the cold arena, steam rising from her reddish coat and a light, frothy drool accumulating on her lower lip, I decide that even though I know only a little about dressage, with its endless complexity, I do know loveliness when I see it.

Before I came to East Hill, almost all my experience with equine loveliness had to do with jumping things, so it's not much of a surprise that, since I have been riding again, I have also been going out of my way to watch horses jump things on television. When I can, anyway: It's surprising how difficult this is to do in the United States. The people in charge of American programming will lavish airtime on bowling, fishing, poker, and dog shows, but show jumping, which is widely broadcast in other parts of the world, is somehow below their collective commercial radar. This neglect continues despite the sport's inherent drama and accessibility—it isn't like golf or baseball, which have long periods of not much happening and rules you really have to know ahead of time. Instead show jumping offers nonstop action, and the scoring is based on the simple premise that knocking down a jump is bad. A secondary premise is that speed is important. If you and your horse can do it quickly and not hit anything, you'll win.

Thoroughbred racing, of course, gets plenty of coverage, and is also based on a very simple concept: The fast horse wins. Sometimes I watch racing, but only for the post parade. I love seeing that line of fillies and colts find their way to the starting gate, their young bodies lustrous and fit, their ears like semaphores, taking in the crowd, the jockey, the footing, and the possible approach of tiger-laden thunderstorms. I particularly like watching these big glossy horses jog alongside the plainer and more placid lead ponies, whose job it is to coax them along quietly to the gate. It's a study in contrast: The ponies (who are rarely actual ponies; they come in various sizes) tend to be foursquare and sensible under their heavy Western tack, unflappable in the presence of a scatty two-year-old. Sometimes the fancy horse and the ordinary one have a brief discussion, bumping noses and shoulders, but for professional reasons it never lasts very long. Lead ponies are all business, as solid and as honorable as tugboats.

I can see the grace of these young Thoroughbreds, absorb their vigor, and appreciate that this is what they are bred to do, but once the horses are in the gate—a tense, interesting transaction—I invariably lose interest. This partly because I have never bet on a racehorse and probably never will, which takes away any fiscal thrill, but my boredom, if that's what it is, is actually more stubborn and untrusting. The outcome of the race always comes too quickly, and the actual logistics of getting to the finish, while no doubt very complicated, don't seem worth it to me. This is an artifact of having seen too many horses come off the track to be re-trained for some other discipline, and too much exposure to what racing can do to the young equine body. There is a wide river of damaged horses limping off the backstretch, bringing with them their bowed tendons and big knees and worrisome X-rays. They are beautiful, ruined babies, asked to do too much too soon.

It can certainly be argued that jumping big, trappy, oddly spaced, and deliberately uninviting fences is also quite hard on horses, and unnatural to boot, but show jumping unfolds differently from the horse and human perspectives. Perhaps because it is unnatural, it is also more selective: Even a pokey racehorse likes to run, if only out of peer pressure and a generic desire to keep up with the action, but a jumper enters the arena alone and with very little obvious incentive to offer a clear round. Some horses take on the physical and mental challenges with pleasure, while others are hassled and upset by them—a jumper who does not like to jump is, by definition, not a jumper. There is a strange and important reason for this: When a horse leaves the ground to clear an obsta-cle, he is actually jumping a memory. His vision, which is designed to spot tigers before they get into biting range, has also endowed him with a surprisingly large triangle of nothingness that extends about six feet in front of him. Thus jumping requires that he hold for a long moment the image of the shape, size, and breadth of the thing he is about to encounter, and he lifts into the air hoping he is right and that no harmful or important detail has escaped him. Not every horse is mentally suited to this intellectual exercise, since it places a demand on him that he isn't really designed to meet; if racing is hard on the body, jumping is hard on the cogni-tion. What's interesting, at least to me, is how many horses do rise to the challenge and even shape its content, as Abbott used to, with an individual and unstoppable commitment. It's hard to know, with horses, where obedience ends and initiative begins, but it's easy to know that when a horse crashes wildly through a fence—a surprisingly rare occurrence—it is not a *dis*obedience. It is because he lost his concentration and forgot where it was.

I have treasured knowing this small, important fact every time I have turned down a line and approached an obstacle; I have a secret belief that knowing it makes me better at making jumps happen. I have even pretended to myself while riding that I can sense the moment of disappearance, that flickering instant when the horse decides he knows, or does not know, what the trajectory of this blind flight will be. I understand that he can still see parts of the fence if it is wide enough—this is why narrow fences are so unnerving to so many otherwise skilled hunters and jumpers—but the essentials of the transaction still haunt me. Each time a horse chooses the risk of midair over the certainty of the ground, we have an obligation to acknowledge that the horse is not *just* jumping. He is navigating according to his own inward imagery.

This fact about jumping is one of the things that makes watching horses jump infinitely variable and infinitely interesting, and I confess I have exasperated more than one companion by my perfect readiness to spend hours on end doing nothing else. Heat, cold, wind, rain, bad footing, hard seats, no seats, dust, sunburn—as Kathie sometimes says, it *doesn't matter*. What matters is watching the turn, the moment when the horse locates and begins to process the next obstacle or combination, and the slender slice of time in which he absorbs what is worth knowing and decides what he will do. Or perhaps not do—a refusal to jump is often formulated while the fence is still visible and the horse, cooking along at ten or twelve miles an hour, decides he cannot or will not find his way over this particular approaching memory. He may need more time, or there may be something about it that alarms him. He may rock back and stiffen or change the way he bends his knees. A good rider can be profoundly reassuring, and can often persuade him to reconsider, but the point is that jumps are not *just* jumps but image-based decisions, often made quickly under stressful circumstances. The weather, the discomfort, the call of other obligations, for me do not enter into it—I feel a duty to watch.

It is very nice, I admit, to watch it on TV from a comfortable couch—the Canadian station that I monitor for its show-jumping programming offers wonderful camera angles, long views, close-ups, slo-mo, and extravagantly good commentary; an international competition with a big field can run an entire afternoon. This is a little like having a bottomless bowl of ice cream, and sometimes I tape the broadcast so I can spoon up the whole thing again later. Knowing which horse-and-rider combination will eventually win doesn't seem to have any effect on my level of interest; in fact, the longer I watch, the more the results seem to recede in importance. Sometimes, as I sprawl on the sofa, I have to sniff away some tears during a particularly beautiful performance that I already know will end in big trouble at the triple combination, a demanding run of jumps that often comes at the exact moment when the horses are getting tired. Even though I did very little of this kind of jumping on Bones—our specialty was the long, hard gallop over banks and timber and the easy lines and inviting obstacles of the hunter ring—the truth is that she could have done it, since she had the show jumper's power, flexibility, and analytic style. I watch the horses go and relive the lift, the snap of her knees, the long parabola of her neck reaching up and over, and that glorious moment when she landed cleanly on the far side of a spectral memory and galloped on—a moment when it was suddenly possible to breathe again. These couch-potato tears are not really of awe or even admiration. What I mainly feel is envy.

Once you have ridden a good jumper, this kind of envy comes easily. Bones was a good one, one of those rare horses who jump reflexively—the question posed by an obstacle, no matter how awkward or intimidating, was always answered with a blank, un-hesitating ease. She interpreted the approach of an obstacle as a sufficient and pure reason to go over it, since this was preferable to going around it. Why her mind worked this way is unknown, since Bones was not a particularly obedient horse, and it can probably be argued that she wasn't a particularly clever one, either. But this un-thinking preference was not stupidity. It was something else, something mysterious to me and often exhilarating. It was as if she were magnetized—she sometimes found herself pulled over ob-stacles unexpectedly because they were in the vicinity and looked jumpable.

This tendency was very pronounced and once nearly got us killed. On a fast conditioning ride—trot, canter, trot, canter—in preparation for a hunter pace event, we suddenly fetched up at the edge of an embankment with some railroad tracks below. Running along beside the tracks were some utility lines. Sadly, from the top of the embankment, these power lines hung at a perfectly reason-able three foot six, and Bones launched herself into the air to clear them. We landed on the tracks, probably fifteen feet below, and even though she was quite surprised by this unusual outcome, she promptly gathered herself and sprang up the embankment on the other side. I went with her, mostly because there was no time to ac-tually fall off, and the whole episode, potentially quite tragic, still lingers in my memory not as stupid, but as somehow necessary.

Horses like this are rare, and there was always a temptation to jump her far too much. I'm not sure why I resisted it except to say that, however much I loved the feel of her underneath me in the air, I actually preferred the complex discussions that could only take place when her feet were closer to the ground. But I did in-dulge in taking her to local hunter shows each summer, where she steadily consumed brush fences, ditches, gates, water jumps, chicken coops, and timber much the way a champion eater goes through blueberry pies. Jumping her was curiously relaxing, since while she was at work over these obstacles she was free of her usual tics, squirms, and affectations, and became instead a self-absorbed display of airborne magnificence. She often placed well in difficult classes against much fancier horse-and-rider combinations, and the only thing that ever darkened the judge's card was her tendency toward excessive speed.

Unfortunately, I came away from the long experience of riding her stuffed to the ears with some very odd assumptions. Over the years, I had mastered perfectly the length of her stride, her preferred distances for takeoff, her way of switching leads to balance herself at the canter, and even which fat, tricolored braid in her mane I could park my fists on in the air—a necessary maneuver, since she was smooth but very powerful, and I often needed something to steady myself against. So I was not all that pleased to discover that most horses were much more work to jump, and did not carry themselves in the same effortless way. But the really big assumption I carried with me was that all horses would of course go over all fences, and that this was not a part of the transaction I needed to worry about. This proved untrue, but the durability of this belief was so strong that many horses I rode later went over many fences, often to their own astonishment, simply because I behaved as if they would. So even though riding, at its core, is a profoundly truthful enterprise, there are still moments when untrue things come in handy.

The art of riding a good horse over a big fence goes well beyond the physical exertion of setting a good line, following the takeoff, and absorbing the landing, mostly because after a while these things become internalized, much the way you internalize how to drive a car with a standard transmission. The mechanics of the thing aside, what you often feel is a pleasurable combination of fear and premature triumph. There's an episode in Somerville and Ross's *Some Experiences of an Irish R.M.* that, however you feel about foxhunting, captures this particular brand of ecstasy. The narrator, Sinclair, who is frankly not much of a rider, finds himself at a local meet where he has been plonked on a strange horse with the ominous name of Sorcerer. It is not a comfortable situation, and takes a turn for the worse when the hunt turns unexpectedly fast and thrilling—many hunts are surprisingly dull, and dullness is clearly what the narrator had been hoping for. As the hounds pull away, Sinclair notes that the other riders respond by taking hold of their horses. "I did likewise," he says, "but with the trifling difference that my horse took hold of me." Barely in control, Sinclair finds himself galloping toward a "stone-faced bank with broken ground in front of it."

> That Sorcerer shortened his stride at the right moment was entirely due to his own judgment. Standing well away from the jump, he rose like a stag out of the tussocky ground, and as he swung my twelve stone six into the air the obstacle revealed itself to him and me as consisting not of one bank but of two, and between the two lay a deep grassy lane, half choked with furze. I have often been asked to state the width of the bohereen, and can only reply that in my opinion it was at least eighteen feet; Flurry Knox and Dr. Hickey, who did not jump it, say that it was not more than five. What Sorcerer did I cannot say; the sensation was of a towering flight with a kickback in it, a biggish drop, and a landing on cee-springs, still on the downhill grade. That was how one of the best horses in Ireland took one of Ireland's most ignorant riders over a very nasty place.

I have often wondered if there is anything quite like this up-and-over sensation of taking a large fence on a trustworthy horse.

Perhaps it's a bit like half-pipe snowboarding, with its hanging aerobatics; perhaps the sheer thrust correlates nicely to being shot out of a cannon. Since I don't snowboard and have not yet run away to join the circus, I can't be sure. What I am sure of is that, even if these airborne moments are alike in degree, they are different in kind, since neither unfolds in the close company of another species, different in a thousand ways from you and me but sharing, for the duration, the sensation of doing something hard and doing it well.

The downside of jumping, of course, is that things can go horribly wrong. The obstacles in the show-jumping ring look solid, but they actually have a lot of potential moving parts; most of these fences are deliberately constructed so that rails come down easily, and even a minor mistake can result in an amazing display of collapsing timber. This is done not to make the competition harder but to make it safer: A fence that dissolves really is an improvement over a fence that is nailed together, as many cross-country obstacles are. Imagine for a moment that Sorcerer had not cleared the double wall with the sunken road in between, and what the consequences might have been for horse and rider, and you will quickly grasp that a huge spread jump—which is essentially what Sinclair's obstacle turned out to be—is better made of wooden rails sitting on flat cups than rocks and mortar. Yet there is always the danger of these rails taking unpredictable trajectories, and a horse in midair is vulnerable to interference. And so is a rider—a sudden disaster or refusal can launch a human headfirst into a jumble of poles, plywood panels, and potted geraniums. The aftermath of this parabola can be unpredictable, as the actor Christopher Reeve, who was paralyzed and eventually died as the result of a jumping accident, proves unambiguously. Almost everyone who takes jumping seriously eventually gets injured—wrists are particularly vulnerable because we instinctively try to use our hands to cushion a fall, and I once knew someone who was dragged after a fence and as a result lost half her eyesight and all her teeth. I have been lucky—I once broke my hand and hurt my knee, and another time I face-planted into a gate and gave myself a magnificent shiner. These are trivial injuries compared to what happened to Superman, but the plain fact is that jumping takes courage.

But even though jumping sometimes sends horses and humans in different, unexpected directions, jumping also brings them into alignment. As is often the case with horses, mapping and spatial matters come into play, since much about riding over fences boils down to the idea of *finding a distance*. This phrase refers to the precise spot on the planet where a particular horse needs to leave the ground to clear a particular fence; on a strictly mechanical level, finding a distance is the calculation of the trajectory required to clear the jump with a little something to spare. As a general principle, this is not hard to understand, since even we two-legged animals find distances when we leap over a brook or a flower bed. We intuitively grasp the arc of jumping and the physics that go with it, and most of us know to our sorrow the consequences of leaving the ground too late or too soon.

So the idea that there is a right place to jump from is not one that people struggle with; the difficulty lies in its practical ramifications while navigating a round of fences. A jump, in essence, is an elevated, distorted, and very exciting canter stride, and, just to make things interesting, it is the elevated and distorted stride of an animal who may have his own ideas about when to leave the ground and whether there are tigers waiting for him on the other side. Dealing with these contingencies takes practice, and one thing you learn quickly about jumping is that it is actually the three or four canter strides before the jump that determine what is going to happen, since they place the horse and rider inside a fairly narrow zone of jumping possibility. The goal is to ride your distance artfully—the canter can roll forward, making up for lost yardage, or shorten down to compensate for a fence that is coming up too soon. The canter can also be finessed to ensure that, when you have two obstacles in proximity, you really do have the right-shaped horse to meet the second element as intended. There are in-and-outs—two jumps with a single canter stride in between—and triples—three jumps in a row—and many other combinations that call for *steady twos* and *easy threes*. Riders talk this way—lines of related jumps are named by their striding counts and probable characteristics. You can hear cryptic-sounding discussions at ringside: "Is that a going four or a steady five?" "For Thunder, that vertical-to-oxer might well be a three." This way of talking is a planning tool, a linguistic vector where the possibilities of stride intersect with the size, placement, spread, building materials, and characteristics of the obstacle, which in turn intersect with the speed, willingness, and personal history of the horse. And so you count: *one* through the in-and-out, *five* between the gate and the hogsback spread, *two* and *two* through the triple combination. It's a kind of chant, an incantation against trouble or disaster, and, sometimes, an incantation against reality. The horse can *chip in*, adding a short stride if his confidence is low, or *get in long* and leave the ground too early, diving at the jump like a harried commuter chasing a receding train. These factual intrusions happen all the time but do not seem to do any lasting damage to the process of finding distances—an attentive rider keeps it up no matter what, making adjustments right up to the moment when the object of all this spatial calculation flickers out of existence for the primary responsible party. The distance must be found—reliably, carefully, and consistently—since finding it, and riding your horse exactly to it, is what separates a good jumping effort from a jerky, awkward, or dangerous one.

Described this way, jumping does sound like more trouble than it's worth, but this is where it quietly merges with dressage and becomes subtle, precise, and intimate. I've always known this, but now it has practical and personal ramifications. Watching the tiny airborne creatures on TV, it's hard not to notice that the best ones have that dressage expression, in that they meet the bridle in that delicate way, their backs rounded and their hind legs well under them. Some of them have the chesty and balanced brightness of Ruth's horses in training; others are as studious as Reba or as cadenced as the late Railund. I wonder at first if the jumpers I remember watching in my twenties and early thirties were somehow different, although I can't see how that could be the case, but then I slowly realize that it's my eye that is starting to change—I am looking for, and seeing, the symptoms of a complete equine education.

As the competition on TV winds down, though, I find that I do not really want to begin jumping again. I could—lots of people at East Hill are doing it, and there seem to be plenty of jumps around—but it now seems a little adolescent, like roughhousing or maybe a water fight. The riding I have been doing recently seems more age-appropriate, more gratifying, and somehow more deeply felt, and makes complicated demands I am unlikely to outgrow. So even though I am still theoretically equal to the physical challenges of jumping, I discover that I no longer have a need to be airborne. What I want, instead, is the kind of riding that unfolds between the fences, full of intimacy and a hundred small adjustments. I can skip the risk of takeoff but still get the satisfaction that jumping brings. I have to wonder if I'm just being a wimp, but I honestly don't think so. What has happened is that I have *found my distance.*

SIXTEEN

AS IF BY MAGIC, I AM RIDING PRINCE AGAIN. IT HAS BEEN NEARLY a year since that first time I groomed him and probably six months since I forsook him and moved on to Dr. Denton, Railund, and Reba, but he still greets me knowingly, lifts his feet eagerly, leans into the dandy brush, and offers his big face for caressing and attention. Which it definitely needs—Prince is as filthy as he always aspires to be, this time with winter mud, so thickly applied that I need to scare up a towel to dig some of it out of his left ear. Once he is presentable and I can climb aboard, he again offers up his rubbery, curiously happy little walk, and its bounce is contagious—I can feel myself relaxing and cheering up. Not that I was sad before, but now I am *on Prince*, which is always a pleasant place to be. Riding him is a little bit like taking a child to a playground or the circus; he feels pleasantly keyed up, eager to get on with things, and ready for fun. The chiaroscuro of the indoor arena, with its yellow lights and dark, springy floor, suddenly seems intimate, friendly, even festive, and not merely what happens every winter when the days become dark and short. Prince proceeds along the track in his best pony imitation of a giraffe, his head in the air and his back hollow underneath my seat. He sniffs the cold air and flutters his nose—not quite snorting, but close—releasing little puffs of humid steam.

The feel of Prince is both familiar and new, since I find I am, at long last, an improved rider. Instead of letting myself get mired in his distractible and rubbery waywardness, I send him forward into it, and Prince offers up his sifting, crooked, and merry little trot. But I do not accept *little*; I ask, repeatedly, that the trot go *big*, a thing I learned from Railund. Prince is mildly distraught by this requirement and tries to appease me by hurrying, so I slow down my posting—the rider's up-and-down movement that helps makes the trot more rhythmic—and use my legs and seat to invite, cajole, and sometimes insist that the trot be less busy and more connected. I also find the corner of his mouth with my outside hand, the one toward the wall, and set up camp there, waiting for the *forward* I learned from Railund to translate into the *flexion* I learned from Reba. It takes a while but it eventually materializes, tentatively at first, and with it comes a slight tingling, an electric sensation. Every horse is different: Where Reba likes to lean and Railund liked to settle, Prince likes to turn into a Christmas toy with a fresh battery or maybe one of those buzzing, upscale toothbrushes. At the same time, something in my elbow, something buried deep in the joint, is talking directly to something specific in Prince's body, and I sense the discussion is taking place both under me and behind me, in what feels like the swing of his hind leg. Prince lowers his head and begins to listen, and I am suddenly riding every angle of this unusually squirmy and opinionated horse.

I can't always sustain this improved connection—I blunder and lose his attention, sometimes I drive too hard, sometimes I catch him with an insensitive aid—but I am still gratified. Instead of the drift and dribble we produced six months ago, we now offer the world brief moments of real cohesion, straightness, and precision; our circles are often true circles, with Prince holding a consistent bend and posture in the bridle, and the circle being an emergent property of this consistency. He feels looser and fuller and his ears go funny, flopping slightly sideways as he trots, and the effect is curiously doglike. He even starts to drool and then foam a little at the lips, a sign that is bad in dogs but very good among horses, proof that he is welcoming and thinking new thoughts about the bit. His back swings with a resilient, bungee-corded freedom; every boxy corner is now soft and rounded.

Kathie does not really notice—she seems to assume that all my results will now be better—and scolds a little when a transition from canter down to trot has Prince double-clutching and falling into a longer and messier frame. "Do that again," she says, "and this time breathe out and keep that inside leg on. Don't let him go backward into trot. You're not slowing him down, you're reshaping his tempo. Don't ease off. It's forward, forward, forward." We do it again, bungle, and do it a third time with a more acceptable result—the new gait reaches brightly, he stays in my hands with that warm, steady humming, and he somehow understands that, when I deepen my seat and exhale, this slow release of air is a legitimate signal.

"Okay, better," Kathie says after this effort, "but I still want you to get on target with him and then really stay there. Hear his answers and make your corrections, but keep them exactly the right size. When things go well, you still want to quit riding, and because you quit things fall apart, and then you have to get in there and do way too much. I want you in there all the time, to keep things from slipping in the first place. I want you right in the middle, doing tiny things, invisible things, keeping connection going. It's your job, not his, to hold together the discussion."

I've heard this correction several hundred times before, and Prince probably agrees with it, but I am secretly pleased by our performance. My last encounter with Prince wasn't really a disaster, but it wasn't a success, either; even though I am still sometimes failing with him, I have an idea that I'm now failing in a more interesting way. Proof of this is that I discover Prince will actually give me a few steps of a movement called travers, or haunches-in, and this puffs me up some. I have recently been doing more and more lateral exercises on Reba, where she is asked to go both forward and sideways at the same time, and I like this kind of riding. So does Reba, and it seems to catch her by surprise that she can do it at all. She's like a kid who has figured out how to shuffle cards like a grown-up, in two arched and expert stages. She waits eagerly for my leg and greets it with stretching, reaching, and—because she is Reba—inquiring. Prince—because he is Prince—approaches the whole sideways business differently. Despite being so flexible, he wants no part of slithering around on cue, and prefers to stick his head in the air and look unhappy. Yet somehow, on the third or fourth try, I coax, breathe, release, and tickle him along into the movement I remember, and he moves on two tracks more than halfway down the long side of the arena. "That's good enough," says Kathie. "It's hard for him. Praise him and we'll call that a wrap."

Driving home in the dark, though, I can feel my warm little ball of self-congratulation slowly cool and harden. It bothers me that my progress is slow, that I know too little, that things are unnecessarily difficult, that getting a few steps of haunches-in on a scrubby buckskin pony is not much of an accomplishment. This mood may be seasonal: I never like it when we approach the dark pivot of the winter solstice, that time John Donne called the year's midnight. More likely, though, it is caused by another thing about riding that is not much talked about but is generically true: It is difficult to improve in a straight line and impossible to improve as fast as you want to. Only in stories do riders transform overnight into what Velvet Brown, in *National Velvet*, prayerfully describes as "the best rider in England." That book, which is the *ur* story about the potent mix of horses and desire, has Velvet conditioning her horse for the Grand National over what appears to be a few scant weeks, and she herself becomes a skilled steeplechase rider who finds her way around a four-mile course of big timber jumps by following the advice of her nonriding ground coach, Mi. He tells her to "keep as still as you can, and put confidence in him." Real riding does not work that way, but in stories it has to—we'd feel thwarted and disappointed if the plotline revealed the setbacks, schooling, time, money, labor, and preparation that are actually involved.

Much about *National Velvet* is evasive in this way, but there is something about its vagueness that is curiously important. The book is full of oblique dialogue and strange, almost grunting transactions, so that the act of reading begins to feel like eavesdropping. Here is a typical exchange, a domestic after-dinner scene:

"Box," said Mr. Brown, indicating the sideboard. Edwina rose and brought him his small cigar.

The shadows whirled.

"Monday," said Mrs. Brown.

"Driving night," said Velvet.

"What I was thinking," said Mrs. Brown. "Get on off!"

"First?" said Velvet.

"First," said Mrs. Brown.

Velvet hunched her shoulder blades and sniffed. Was driving worth it? She could never make up her mind. Out of bed it didn't seem so, but in bed it was worth while.

It is not until much later that we learn what this scrap of dialogue is really about—Velvet has assigned herself nights for certain types of equine fantasy play, and on Mondays she drives the carriage—but by the time we know this, the exchange has been forgotten, lost in the fugue state that characterizes the entire story. This is not necessarily an authorial affectation, done to puzzle the reader or add to the work of decipherment. Instead it is actually writing of a very high order, the kind that coalesces from the dense air that breathes and circulates within the world of this story. It is no accident, for example, that the final race and Velvet's triumph actually unfold in a sudden and impenetrable fog, so that we never see her or her piebald horse jump a single obstacle. This is strange—the blindness of jumping carried to some weird extreme—but it is also exactly what the author intended. She didn't need to summon the fog, and, having done so, she could easily have narrated events from Velvet's point of view. Instead the account of the Grand National is given by Mi, who spends most of the race running around, hampered by the crowd and the spectral weather conditions, anxiously asking everyone what is going on.

There was a struggle going on at Becher's [a large ditch-and-drop jump]; a horse had fallen and was being got out with ropes. Mi's legs turned to water and he asked his neighbor gruffly, "Who's fallen?" But the neighbor, straining to the tip of his toes, and glued to his glasses, was as deaf as lead. . . . There was a shout and a horse, not riderless, but ridden by a tugging, cursing man, came galloping back through the curling fumes of the mist, rolled its wild eye at the wrong side of Becher's and disappeared away out of the course. An uproar began along the fringes of the crowd and rolled back to where Mi stood. Two more horses came back and rolled out of the mist, one riderless. The shades of others could be discerned in the fog. Curses rapped out from unseen mouths.

"What's happened at the Canal Turn? What's wrong down at the Turn?"

"The whole field!" shouted a man. The crowd took it up.

"The field's out. The whole field's come back. There's no race!"

Of course there *is* a race, with its foregone conclusion, but the chaos and poor visibility go well beyond the demands of having a bit of suspense. In truth, the whole book is suffused with dreams that veer into nightmare, so much so that almost all of Velvet's important contact with The Piebald takes place in her sleep. Before she wins him in a raffle with a borrowed shilling, this four-legged escape artist is signified chiefly by the nighttime clatter of hooves outside her bedroom window; once she acquires him, she dreams vividly of jumping him off a high cliff into the sea. I am not nitpicking. Quite the opposite. The book is important not in spite of this oblique, dreamy quality, but because of it. Deep in the fog of sleep, the heroine subverts the supposedly normal girlish yearnings for jewelry into an aesthetic longing for horse equipment: "Snaffles and straights and pelhams and twisted pelhams were hanging, jointed and still in the shadows of a stable. . . . On her left and right were open stalls made of dark wood and the buttocks of the bay horses shone like mahogany all the way down." When she wakes groggily to the harpylike caterwauling of her sister's canaries, who "screamed in a long yellow scream, and grew madder," she hears outside her windows the passing of the invisible runaway horse, spectral and enticing.

It's a strange household: Downstairs, the Brown family is blessed and burdened with Donald, the youngest child, who is full of gnomic pronouncements, and with Jacob, a fox terrier so dishonest, fawning, and obsequious as to perhaps qualify as one of the great animal portraits in literature. Spaniels lean against the front door, perpetually yearning for admittance, and collapse through it like sacks of grain every time it is opened; another dog, described only as "black" and "barking," lives somewhere outside on a string. "This dog had a name but no character. It barked without ceasing day and night. Nobody heard it. The Browns slept and lived and ate beside its barking." At night, one of Velvet's sisters calls out for Africa, which is not a place but a bird who has died, an event that has offered the reader an affecting if miniature expiration scene; the older Brown sisters, who meet all the fairy-tale requirements for beauty, are beyond beautiful—they are "greyhounds." The boundary between the animal world and the human one is deliberately blurred with an excess of dreaming; it is dreaming, in the end, that allows Velvet to capture her final victory.

National Velvet was written in 1935 and set the bar for all the necessary elements of a good horse story—pluck, virtue, redemption, good fortune against high odds, and the triumph of childlike and ungrasping ambition. I especially like it because the equine hero in it is spotted—once you have owned a carousel horse, they have permanent appeal—and I was confused, when I saw the movie version, to see that "The Piebald" was cast as an ordinary and orthodox chestnut. But *National Velvet* is also a dark story, and after my session with Prince I seem to sink into this darkness—there are times when the price of being the best rider seems too high. Readers often forget, once the story is over, that Velvet set the plot in motion when she "saw the new moon. She bowed three times, glanced round to see that no one saw, then standing in the shadow of the stable door she put her hands like thin white arrows together and prayed to the moon—'Oh God, give me horses, give me horses!' "

This prayer is answered not with the drawing of the fateful raffle ticket—that episode comes later—but with a suicide. Early one morning, Velvet is sent to a neighboring farm, the Cellini estate, with a meat delivery—her father is a butcher—and when she gets there she encounters the Cellini patriarch in the garden, standing by a tree. He behaves very strangely, asking her a lot of disconnected questions; when offered the meat, he throws it away. After a series of unsettling exchanges, he asks her, "Would you tell me what you want most in the world? Would you tell me that?"

"Horses," she said, "sir."

"To ride on? To own for yourself?"

He was still looking at her, as though he expected more.

"I tell myself stories about horses," she went on, desperately fishing at her shy desires. "Then I can dream about them. Now I dream about them every night. I want to be a famous rider, I should like to carry dispatches. I should like to get a first at Olympia; I should like to ride in a great race; I should like to have so many horses that I could walk down between the two rows of loose boxes and ride what I chose. I would have them all under fifteen hands. I like chestnuts best, but bays are lovely too, but I don't like blacks."

Cellini agrees with her that the smaller horses are often the nicest, and then shows Velvet around his stable, introducing her to his saddle horses and telling each one's history—the jumper, the polo pony, the child's hack, the cob, the unbroken filly. Once the tour is over, he sits down and draws out a sheet of paper, begins writing, and then calls for witnesses, in this case the groom and the gardener's boy. He signs the document and then stands up and puts his overcoat over his arm. "Take that paper," he says to Velvet, "and you stay here." Having now written his will, he steps around the corner of the yard and shoots out his brains; Velvet, who a few pages back had prayed to the moon for horses, has suddenly inherited more horses than she knows what to do with. It's magical and gratifying, but it's also emotionally expensive and grotesque.

Riding, it seems to me during the icy drive homeward, really is a form of prayer: Lord, give me horses. As prayers go, it's a good one, an equine *paternoster* of forgiveness and deliverance, but there are other times, like now, when it is painful. I want perfection and validation from Prince, and perhaps a transforming kiss, but that is not how things are going to happen. The fog on the course at the Grand National, and everything it implies, is a denial of the changeable and unforgiving climate around actual, troublesome, in-dividual horses, where *keeping still* and *putting confidence in them* is not adequate or legitimate instruction. Thus the redemption of the fic-tional Piebald, à la *National Velvet*, can be pretty discouraging when you have tried to redeem a real one. In the time it takes me to cover the nine slippery miles home to Montpelier, my sympathy slides away from Velvet and toward Cellini, with his hard, adult questions about what it is we desire. He reminds us that our yearnings are, by necessity, a form of tragedy, and then disappears around the corner of the story with his coat folded neatly on his arm.

SEVENTEEN

NATIONAL VELVET ASIDE, TAKING A TRAGIC VIEW OF HORSES ONLY works intermittently, and the horses themselves never bother with it. Horses feel many things, but most of these feelings are not very sophisticated; tragedy requires reflection and taking a longer, more human view. Plus most horses, if not isolated, are surprisingly game and cheerful, and as if to prove this Reba tells me a joke—perhaps her first one—on a leaden and miserably cold January evening.

I had gotten into the habit of bringing my own grooming kit to the barn. I didn't really need to, since obviously there are brushes there, but many of them are high mileage, splayed as a used toothbrush, and a little rough on Reba's twitchy Thoroughbred skin. So now I bring along my collection of softer, newer brushes, and this importation of my own tools has revived an old habit of sometimes letting the horse look at and sniff each item before I use it. I am clueless where this little ritual comes from; I think I have always done it. With this particular encounter, though, and perhaps as a way of distracting herself from the cold, Reba really inspects each item as I offer it, snuffling hard and wiggling her ears. She seems interested. When I get to the final stage, where I add some shine by running an old towel over her, she sniffs the proffered square of terry cloth, nips it up, flaps it a few times, and then gives it back to me.

"There you go," I tell her. "Good girl."

It's always hard to judge the status of some unprompted new behavior, but her alert posture tells me this is probably meant to be commentary, and perhaps amusing commentary at that. Some horses chew on things the way humans chew on gum or pencils, and many horses nibble inquisitively at pockets and hands, hoping for a treat, but Reba has never been inclined this way; the one time I offered her part of an apple, she was hesitant and surprised and almost rejected it. Because she is not a nibbler, this flapping feels and looks like play—on some wordless, equine level, she's joshing with me. I think about the vigilant and overcautious horse she was when she came to the barn last summer, and how unlikely she would have been, back then, to indulge in jest, and it's another tiny indicator that things are continuing to move in the right direction. Another is that her girth barely fits her—the hot bubbly lungs inside her rib cage are expanding, and she continues to gain weight.

For reasons that have never been adequately explained, ponies, like Prince, have more jokes in them than horses, like Reba. Prince, for example, would certainly find a way to subvert what I do next, which is to select four soft, clean leg wraps from the windowsill in the tack room and begin bandaging Reba's legs—a procedure she accepts without comment and perfectly understands. I know, though, that wrapping Prince's lumpy yellow legs would turn quickly into slapstick, and the final job would be a loose, sloppy mess. This is not because I cannot wrap a horse, but because Prince would clown around and deflect my desire for tidiness, and the finished bandages would droop like knee socks on a child who fell in the frog pond on the way home from school.

Ponies do this, and many other things, and nobody knows why. They undo latches, chase puppies, spill water, scatter their shoes, chew mittens, and butt you with their bony heads; I once had a school pony who began the evening in a box stall and turned up the next morning in a screened breezeway, having liberated a pig somewhere along the way. I spent most of the forenoon trying to catch him, only to have him return to the barn of his own accord when the hay truck came. Since I now had to wrangle bales and had no time for him, the whole business of being loose was no longer a particularly sporting proposition, so he whiled away the time by chewing up the walls of the indoor arena. I have heard stories about angelic ponies, but I am not sure I really believe them. I suppose it's possible that these ponies may be truly and deeply good, the way a horse can choose to be, but it is equally possible that they are biding their time, scouting the horizon for a really good opportunity.

Tonight Reba's legs are cool and hard, but I bandage her anyway—Kathie once said she suspects her circulation isn't all that good, and I think she's right. If Reba doesn't get enough turnout, her hind fetlocks puff up a little, so that when I touch them I can make a brief indent with my fingers—not deep, but enough to worry over. She's also a Florida horse, and this is her first winter in the Vermont cold; keeping her comfortable has been challenging. It does not take a very big leap of imagination to believe that the warming bandages, correctly applied, probably feel pretty good.

It also does me good to apply them. The leg wraps at East Hill are made of a soft, feltlike, flannelly substance, and there is a real trick to doing a good job. You have to start the process properly by angling the first few inches of the fabric upward, at forty-five degrees, and making the first turn so that a triangle—the edge of the start of the roll—sticks up above the first pass of bandage, just below the knee. You then have to fold this triangle down and secure it with an extra pass so that the wrap doesn't loosen from the inside. It's a deft thing to do, like making a hospital corner on a bed. It also takes practice to know exactly how much pressure to apply (snug but not tight) and to get the right amount of overlap per bandage pass (a third the width) so that you can go all the way down the cannon bone, over the fetlock, and reach exactly halfway up the cannon bone again before you run out of material. Then you can uncurl the frizzy little band of male Velcro and reach it around to meet the female band of Velcro that is sewn strategically into the last six inches of the bandage. The genders meet with that Velcro kiss, something between a crackle and a sigh. This sound is serious and sporty—it evokes wrist braces, ski clothing, bulletproof vests— and it's hard not to meditate for a moment on whoever it was who positioned these tapes just so, and whoever it was who decided exactly how long this particular wrap should be, and the amount of planning that went on behind the scenes so that Reba's legs could be kept warm on a day when the temperature is barely above zero.

It occurs to me as I do this that it has now been exactly a year since that first time I was sent to catch Prince, slipping through the snow in the winter sunshine, and I celebrate this anniversary by noting that everything in my life is at once exactly the same and completely changed. I go to the same job, sleep in the same ratty pajamas, write checks off the same bank account, and feel the same contentment when I pull into the home place in the evening and see that Vince is there ahead of me and the lights are on. Yet I am not the same. I am happier and less frightened, I am not mad at anybody, and parts of my past now make much more sense to me. A lot has happened: I am a better rider, even if only marginally so; I have more to think about and frame these thoughts with more intensity; I have looked at horses and allowed those horses to look back at me. I have reclaimed my interest in a certain kind of drama, witnessing the horse-world versions of weddings, graduations, and funerals.

What I mostly feel, though, is that I am a less trivial human being, and, because of this, I feel an obligation to doubt my motives. Am I here in this cold aisle, wrapping Reba's second foreleg, because I secretly want to be young again? Because for the most part I really don't—to be young, to a large degree, is to be strong but stupid, blissfully unaware of the dangers of gum disease. But I can't be completely sure about this. When Bones died, I assumed wrongly that I could close the book on my various youthful horse adventures, that I'd done a good-enough job at what I had set out to do, which was to approximate her redemption. But the book refused to close all the way, and I kept a clumsy finger in between the pages, going on to own two more horses who, to be perfectly honest, I never found all that interesting. One was earnest but chronically lame; the other, the Thoroughbred filly, was irredeemably conventional, despite my many efforts to figure out what she liked to do. These horses bored me—I think we bored each other—and this was discouraging. Two flops in a row did seem like a signal that I was past it, and so I came to believe that something truly ended on that autumn afternoon when Bones folded her knees and lay down, shoulders first, haunches second, and then went over on her side. I wasn't there, but I'm guessing she probably kicked a little, because dying horses always do, and her big, worried, and complicated heart stopped beating. She was thirty-four, and except for that bit of spavin, still sound, but she had lost interest in the world and had simply stopped eating. The vet's injection meant that she could die quietly, which was not at all how she had lived. It wasn't sad so much as empty. My mother called a local contractor with a backhoe and we buried her.

When I hold the wrap between my palms and test it, it's slightly loose, and loose won't do—it may come unraveled during work, and it won't give Reba the support she needs. I unwrap, reroll, and begin again. As I progress again down the mare's patient leg, I think about how, even after a horse has been buried, the story that died with her can still appear in unexpected syndication. Once reactivated, it then demands continual rewinding—not to pretty up the truth, but mostly to see the good horse take the big jump once again. These jumps matter, since they offer both a real and metaphorical change in elevation: Horses, especially the good ones, really do send their humans upward, into the thin air of a different moral plane. The literature of horses—the hundreds of different stories that are all essentially the same—tries hard to explain this, but it is the target of other kinds of writing as well: Hemingway wondered about the carcass of the leopard on the slopes of Kilimanjaro—"No one has explained what the leopard was seeking at that altitude"—and Jon Krakauer, in *Into the Wild*, talks about the inner state that drives mountain climbers endlessly toward the summit. "It is easy," he says, "when you are young, to believe that what you desire is no less than what you deserve, to assume that if you want something badly enough, it is your God-given right to have it." He rapidly acknowledges that this kind of youthful thinking is "obscure" and "gap-ridden," which is certainly true, but he actually goes one useful step beyond that. "I thought," he says, "that climbing the Devil's Thumb would fix all that was wrong with my life. But I came to appreciate that mountains make poor receptacles for dreams."

As I begin on the next leg, it is obvious to me to me that horses make unusually good ones, and that the gappy, obscure logic of youth has nothing to do with it. Quite the opposite. The past year has shown me that my life with horses has actually filled those gaps. I will never ride as well as Ruth or have the incisive and exact teaching skills of Kathie, but I will always have tigers, stillness, attention, willingness, and the weight and the content of now. For example, I can see that now this third leg is going swimmingly—the even lapstrake of the bandage makes a neat turn around the ball of Reba's ankle—and as I find my way back up the bone, I know I will have the exact amount of wrapping needed for a secure and unhurried ending.

Testing the fit, I realize why it can't be a yearning-for-youth thing: My foster parents, now both in their eighties, still ride—my mother has a righteous and bouncy little Paso Fino, a real pony's pony, and my father has a rangy buckskin who looks a lot like Prince, but a Prince who got hung on the line instead of put in the dryer. I'm sure they would both like to be younger—old age hurts—but the excesses of youth now mostly annoy them. At one point, we of the younger generation talked about getting them cell phones to take with them on their trail rides, just in case something bad happened in the woods, but this never came to pass. Maybe a cell phone seemed a little too urban and newfangled, but it's also perfectly possible that we kids—now all in our fifties—are finally old enough to understand that a life with horses offers a perfect balance of benefits and dangers. This may be a false understanding—I think of Ruth hanging horribly in midair, too high for her own good, but I also think of what happened after she landed, and her insistence that she would heal, that she had to, that she was headed for the Olympics. Of course my parents are headed only for the same trails and fields that I once rode through—the surreal tree nursery, the narrow path beside the pond that can sometimes get icy—but there is a touch of Ruth in them or they would not be doing it.

Reba's last leg begins well, but my fingers are getting numb. That I am squatting in an aisle doing something barehanded on a cold winter night is a fact that interests me. It seems like a kind of self-punishment, like something abnormal and perhaps fanatical, but it's exactly what I want to do. What does it mean, I wonder again, when we say that someone has gone *horse crazy*? Velvet Brown certainly had this form of insanity—before getting any real horses, she had a full stable of paper ones that she cupped in her hands as she cantered on two legs across the countryside, tapping her own thigh with a little stick. She looked pretty dorky doing this, and looked dorkier still lying in bed with a cord looped over her toes, pulling these makeshift reins and saying *Careful through the gate. Mind now. Get on, Satin!* My parents, I am quite sure, do not do this, but all around me young girls skitter around the aisles with their buckets and wheelbarrows, their faces glad and serious, and I wonder if any of them ever indulge in these kinds of giddyup fantasies. I certainly did; I used to set up little jumps in the back-yard and prance around, sometimes running out or refusing, some-times surprising myself with a clear round. It was a weird game, since I myself was never quite sure what I was going to do as I can-tered toward an obstacle, and finding out was part of the game's fascination, its mystery. Even then, I had a vestigial awareness of the need for uncertainty, and it was good preparation for the un-certainty of things to come; this may go an inch or two toward ex-plaining why we play these games at all. I don't think bowlers or skiers or golfers do this. I have an idea they actually go bowling, skiing, or golfing instead.

Horse craziness has certain magical, reiterative properties— properties that may be good evidence that riding really does ap-proach spiritual allegory. The stories certainly insist that this is so, even though, as I've come to see, these stories are wrong in many of their particulars. But as Kathie says it *doesn't matter*, since these stories also carry the reader toward redemption—horses achieve greatness, wrongs are righted, and virtue is restored. Still, it seems unlikely that allegory, all by itself, does the trick, since the past year, while carrying all the usual redemptive themes, also brought with it grief, love, work, and endless correction. These are good, hard, useful things, the opposite of allegory, and come bathed in the even light of authenticity. In some basic way, they are *horse* things, even *horse crazy* things, that hold their magic because they refuse to turn into blurry abstractions.

Perhaps these horse things keep their sharp edges, in part, because they are linked to power. Not the Freudian kind, which I think of as controlling and intrusive and essentially masculine, but a different kind of power that I have an idea many women crave and understand. It is power unwielded. As I unroll the soft lengths of flannel around Reba, I am humbled by her strength and courtesy, by her ability to squash me flat and her ongoing decision not to. This is domestication operating, but the arrangement is provisional; with horses, there is always an element of condescension. The power is theirs, but they will loan it, and I like this in some specific, female way. Horses, it seems to me, know how to relinquish power without being diminished, and there is something important and instructive here, something to be grasped, something to be sustained and labored for. It could be that girls and women yearn for horses because horses, on some level, show us what to do. From them, we learn how to avoid too much compromise, watch for predators, get home safely, soar with our eyes closed, and remain beautiful indefinitely. These things offer a coating of spiritual preservative against a corrosive world.

My bandages are done and I come out of my deep-knee bend slowly and creakily, making that little *uh* of exertion that arrives automatically at a certain age. I still need to bridle her but Reba is basically ready, so I assemble the necessities—helmet, gloves, stick—and put a couple of clean tissues in my pocket. I then put my glasses in my grooming bag—they steam up in the cold air of the arena—and hang the bag on a high hook out of the way. I fetch my bridle and slip it over Reba's tulip ears, and at this moment a few of the young girls of East Hill begin to sing along to a pop song on the radio, sweetly and discordantly, very slightly out of key. Prince makes a brief appearance as he is moved from one stall to another so that his grubby, dug-up outhouse of a room can be mucked out, and his fit golden body, as tight and enticing as a sausage, shimmers in the lights as he crosses the aisle. He does not notice me—he is busy with the girls, the singing, and some sort of treat, probably an apple, which he chews with intense conviction. Perhaps what matters is that I notice him, and it may all be this simple: I am glad he exists, and was engaged in conversation with me. The girls are still singing. The song is about love and I linger until it's over, which means that I must hurry now, or I will be late for my lesson.